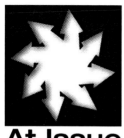

At Issue

How Far Should Science Extend the Human Lifespan?

Other Books in the At Issue Series:

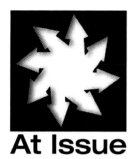

At Issue

How Far Should Science Extend the Human Lifespan?

Tamara Thompson, Book Editor

GREENHAVEN PRESS
A part of Gale, Cengage Learning

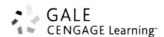

Detroit • New York • San Francisco • New Haven, Conn • Waterville, Maine • London

GALE
CENGAGE Learning™

Christine Nasso, *Publisher*
Elizabeth Des Chenes, *Managing Editor*

© 2009 Greenhaven Press, a part of Gale, Cengage Learning.

Gale and Greenhaven Press are registered trademarks used herein under license.

For more information, contact:
Greenhaven Press
27500 Drake Rd.
Farmington Hills, MI 48331-3535
Or you can visit our Internet site at gale.cengage.com

Articles in Greenhaven Press anthologies are often edited for length to meet page requirements. In addition, original titles of these works are changed to clearly present the main thesis and to explicitly indicate the author's opinion. Every effort is made to ensure that Greenhaven Press accurately reflects the original intent of the authors. Every effort has been made to trace the owners of copyrighted material.

Cover image © Images.com/Corbis.

LIBRARY OF CONGRESS CATALOGING-IN-PUBLICATION DATA

How far should science extend the human lifespan? / Tamara Thompson, editor.
p. cm. -- (At issue)
Includes bibliographical references and index.
ISBN 978-0-7377-4304-3 (hardcover)
ISBN 978-0-7377-4303-6 (pbk.)
1. Longevity. I. Thompson, Tamara.
RA776.75.H863 2009
612.6'8--dc22

2008051756

Printed in the United States of America
2 3 4 5 6   13 12 11 10 09

ED352

Contents

Introduction

People live longer today than at any time in history, thanks to improved living conditions and advances in medical care. In 1900, average life expectancy in the United States was just 47 years; today it is more than 77 years. But that could be just the beginning. *Guinness World Records* recognizes Jeanne Calment of France as the oldest person whose age can be verified. She was 122 years and 124 days old when she died in 1997. But if biomedical researchers are right, that record won't stand much longer, and it could soon be common to live that long—or even much longer.

The booming field of life-extension science primarily focuses on ways to slow, stop, or reverse the aging process. Genetic engineering, calorie-restricted diets, and regenerative cellular medicine are just a few of the avenues of research that promise to add years or decades to the natural human lifespan (now assumed to be less than 130 years). While most aging researchers agree that routinely extending life by ten or twenty years will be soon within the reach of modern science, some are convinced that doubling the natural human lifespan is possible. Still others believe that life can be much more dramatically extended—perhaps indefinitely.

Radical life-extension researcher Aubrey de Grey is arguably the most controversial and extreme of the "prolongevists," those who advocate the development of life-extension technologies. De Grey maintains that because aging is the underlying cause of diseases that lead to death, aging itself should be viewed as a disease that can be cured. De Grey believes that if medical science can stop the damage that aging does to the body's cells, older adults will not develop diseases and the aging process could be effectively stopped. If science can halt the cellular changes caused by aging, de Grey believes humans could routinely live to be 1,000 years old or more. In this radical view of life extension, life could continue indefinitely as long as the body is regularly maintained, much as people now maintain antique cars to keep them in running order. While mainstream scientists tend to write off the eccentric and charismatic de Grey as a crackpot, no one has yet been able to disprove his theories scientifically.

Other life-extension advocates take a comparatively more conservative approach, focusing on improving quality of life and achieving longevity gains that are measured in years and decades rather than centuries. As aging researcher Robert Binstock has noted, the primary goal of life extension should be "adding life to years, not just years to life." That means finding ways to keep people healthy and mobile later into their lives, while at the same time extending their overall lifespans. Even so, many researchers consider doubling the human lifespan to be eventually feasible, if not inevitable.

Regardless of what turns out to be possible at the hand of science, even more controversial is whether greatly extended lifespans would even be desirable or ethical. For many in the prolongevity camp, extending life is a moral imperative. John Harris, a bioethicist at the University of Manchester in England, is one of many who believe that science has a moral duty to extend the human lifespan as far as possible. "When you save a life, you are simply postponing death to another point," Harris says. "Thus, we are committed to extending life indefinitely if we can, for the same reasons that we are committed to life-saving."

Critics of life extension, however, argue that any dramatic gain in life expectancy could have far-reaching and devastating consequences worldwide. They warn of profound demographic shifts as the old make up an ever larger percentage of the population; resource scarcity as demand grows for limited global supplies of water, food, and energy; social strain between generations as they navigate redefined social structures; economic strife as the old compete with the young for jobs throughout their longer working lives; health care inequality as the rich are able to afford life-extension medicine and the poor cannot; political entrenchment as the tenure of world leaders lengthens along with their lifespans; and even psychological and spiritual distress as people grapple with new questions of purpose, destiny, and fulfillment as they live to unprecedented ages.

In the United States, an additional consideration is the aging of the baby boom generation, the seventy-six million people born between 1946 and 1964. The boomers are the nation's largest demographic group, and the first members of this massive cohort have already entered their 50s; the last will turn 55 in 2019. By 2030, roughly 20 percent of the population will be over 65, compared to less than 13 percent right now. Boomers have long played a lead role in shaping American culture, and as they age they are expected to be the most active and healthy older generation the planet has seen. As they transform what it means to grow old, many boomers like to say that "80 is the new 60." With growing access to life-extending technologies, 150 could one day be the new 80. The authors in *At Issue: How Far Should Science Extend the Human Lifespan?* represent a wide range of viewpoints concerning the ethics, practicalities, and consequences of developing and using life-extension technologies.

1

Life Extension: An Overview

Ker Than

Ker Than is a staff writer for LiveScience, a science-oriented Internet content provider.

Humans have long sought a way to extend life and preserve youth and health. Modern science may soon be able to extend healthy life by several decades, which would have far-reaching social implications. A doubled lifespan, for example, would change the way families interact, the way people view their careers, even how they perceive political events and wars. There are also many moral and ethical concerns about life extension. Many experts worry about unfairness emerging between rich and poor, and young and old as they compete for both everyday resources and life-extending technologies. If everyone lives longer, global overpopulation also would become a serious issue. Although there are many benefits of longer life, there are also many disadvantages that must be considered seriously before science enters this new territory.

Adam and Eve lost it, alchemists tried to brew it, and if you believe the legends, Spanish conquistador Juan Ponce de Leon was searching for it when he discovered Florida.

To live forever while preserving health and retaining the semblance and vigor of youth is one of humanity's oldest and most elusive goals.

Now, after countless false starts and disappointments, some scientists say we could finally be close to achieving lifetimes that are, if not endless, at least several decades longer. This modern miracle, they say, will come not from revitalizing waters or transmuted substances, but from a scientific understanding of how aging affects our bodies at the cellular and molecular levels.

If scientists could create a pill that let you live twice as long while remaining free of infirmities, would you take it?

Whether through genetic tinkering or technology that mimics the effects of caloric restriction—strategies that have successfully extended the lives of flies, worms and mice—a growing number of scientists now think that humans could one day routinely live to 140 years of age or more.

Extreme optimists such as Aubrey de Grey think the maximum human lifespan could be extended indefinitely, but such visions of immortality are dismissed by most scientists as little more than science fiction.

While scientists go back and forth on the feasibility of slowing, halting or even reversing the aging process, ethicists and policymakers have quietly been engaged in a separate debate about whether it is wise to actually do so.

A Doubled Lifespan

If scientists could create a pill that let you live twice as long while remaining free of infirmities, would you take it?

If one considers only the personal benefits that longer life would bring, the answer might seem like a no-brainer: People could spend more quality time with loved ones; watch future generations grow up; learn new languages; master new musical instruments; try different careers or travel the world.

But what about society as a whole? Would it be better off if life spans were doubled? The question is one of growing relevance, and serious debate about it goes back at least a few years to the Kronos Conference on Longevity Health Sciences in Arizona.

Gregory Stock, director of the Program on Medicine, Technology and Society at UCLA's [University of California, Los Angeles] School of Public Health, answered the question with an emphatic "Yes."

A doubled lifespan, Stock said, would "give us a chance to recover from our mistakes, lead us toward longer-term thinking and reduce health care costs by delaying the onset of expensive diseases of aging. It would also raise productivity by adding to our prime years."

If we were 100 years younger than our parents or 60 years apart from our siblings, that would certainly create a different set of social relationships.

Bioethicist Daniel Callahan, a co-founder of the Hastings Center in New York, didn't share Stock's enthusiasm. Callahan's objections were practical ones. For one thing, he said, doubling life spans won't solve any of our current social problems.

"We have war, poverty, all sorts of issues around, and I don't think any of them would be at all helped by having people live longer," Callahan said in a recent telephone interview. "The question is, 'What will we get as a society?' I suspect it won't be a better society."

Others point out that a doubling of the human life span will affect society at every level. Notions about marriage, family and work will change in fundamental ways, they say, as will attitudes toward the young and the old.

Marriage and Family

Richard Kalish, a psychologist who considered the social effects of life extension technologies, thinks a longer lifespan will radically change how we view marriage.

In today's world, for example, a couple in their 60s who are stuck in a loveless but tolerable marriage might decide to stay together for the remaining 15 to 20 years of their lives out of inertia or familiarity. But if that same couple knew they might have to suffer each other's company for another 60 or 80 years, their choice might be different.

Kalish predicted that as life spans increase, there will be a shift in emphasis from marriage as a lifelong union to marriage as a long-term commitment. Multiple, brief marriages could become common.

New Types of Generation Gaps

A doubled life span will reshape notions of family life in other ways, too, says Chris Hackler, head of the Division of Medical Humanities at the University of Arkansas.

If multiple marriages become the norm, as Kalish predicts, and each marriage produces children, then half-siblings will become more common, Hackler points out. And if couples continue the current trend of having children beginning in their 20s and 30s, then eight or even 10 generations might be alive simultaneously, Hackler said.

Furthermore, if life extension also increases a woman's period of fertility, siblings could be born 40 or 50 years apart. Such a large age difference would radically change the way siblings or parents and their children interact with one other.

"If we were 100 years younger than our parents or 60 years apart from our siblings, that would certainly create a different set of social relationships," Hackler told LiveScience.

The Workplace

For most people, living longer will inevitably mean more time spent working. Careers will necessarily become longer, and the retirement age will have to be pushed back, not only so individuals can support themselves, but to avoid overtaxing a nation's social security system.

Advocates of anti-aging research say that working longer might not be such a bad thing. With skilled workers remaining in the workforce longer, economic productivity would go up. And if people got bored with their jobs, they could switch careers.

But such changes would carry their own set of dangers, critics say.

The loss of a child and the passing of an elderly person are not the same thing at all. . . . The first is premature, while the latter comes, hopefully, at the end of a well-lived life.

Competition for jobs would become fiercer as "midlife retrainees" beginning new careers vie with young workers for a limited number of entry-level positions.

Especially worrisome is the problem of workplace mobility, Callahan said.

"If you have people staying in their jobs for 100 years, that is going to make it really tough for young people to move in and get ahead," Callahan explained. "If people like the idea of delayed gratification, this is going to be a wonderful chance to experience it."

Callahan also worries that corporations and universities could become dominated by a few individuals if executives, managers and tenured professors refuse to give up their posts. Without a constant infusion of youthful talent and ideas, these institutions could stagnate.

Hackler points out that the same problem could apply to politics. Many elected officials have term limits that prevent them from amassing too much power. But what about federal judges, who are appointed for life?

"Justices sitting on the bench for a hundred years would have a powerful influence on the shape of social institutions," Hackler writes.

Time to Act

A 2003 staff working paper drawn up by the U.S. President's Council of Bioethics—then headed by Leon Kass, a longtime critic of attempts to significantly extend the human lifespan—stated that anti-aging advances would redefine social attitudes toward the young and the old, and not in good ways.

"The nation might commit less of its intellectual energy and social resources to the cause of initiating the young, and more to the cause of accommodating the old," the paper stated. Also, quality of life might suffer. "A world that truly belonged to the living would be very different and perhaps a much diminished world, focused too narrowly on maintaining life and not sufficiently broadly on building the good life."

While opinions differ wildly about what the ramifications for society will be if the human life span is extended, most ethicists agree that the issue should be discussed now, since it might be impossible to stop or control the technology once it's developed.

"If this could ever happen, then we'd better ask what kind of society we want to get," Callahan said. "We had better not go anywhere near it until we have figured those problems out."

Would Immortality Be Ethical?

For John Harris, saving a life and delaying its end [are] one and the same. Using this logic, Harris, a bioethicist at the University of Manchester, England, figures that scientists have a moral duty to extend the human life span as far as it will go, even if it means creating beings that live forever.

"When you save a life, you are simply postponing death to another point," Harris told LiveScience. "Thus, we are committed to extending life indefinitely if we can, for the same reasons that we are committed to life-saving."

But the loss of a child and the passing of an elderly person are not the same thing at all, says Daniel Callahan, a bioethicist at the Hastings Center in New York. The first is premature, while the latter comes, hopefully, at the end of a well-lived life.

Aging research could have a far greater impact on improving public health than trying to cure diseases individually.

"The death of an elderly person is sad, because we lose them and they lose us, but it's not tragic," Callahan said. "One can't say this is a deranged universe to live in because people die of old age."

This is just one of several ethical and moral arguments that have cropped up in recent years as labs around the world aim at the dream of immortality, or at least to extend lives well beyond the century mark. Among other debates:

- Will everyone have an equal chance to drink from a fountain of youth?

- If people live longer but are miserable for decades, will views on suicide and euthanasia change?

- In an immortal society, how do you make room for new generations?

A World of 112-Year-Olds

The life expectancy for the average American is 77.6 years. Extending life spans will be an incremental process, most experts say. But there is great promise.

A 1990 study by University of Chicago biodemographer Jay Olshansky and colleagues calculated that even if the risk of death from cancer in the United States were reduced to zero, average life expectancy would increase by only 2.7 years. If the risks from heart disease, stroke and diabetes were also eliminated, life expectancy would increase by another 14 years, the researchers found.

In contrast, repeated experiments have shown rodents fed 40 percent fewer calories live about 40 percent longer. For reasons that are unclear, this "caloric restriction" regimen also postpones the onset of many degenerative diseases normally associated with aging.

If these effects can be replicated in humans, the average person could live to be 112 years old and our maximum life span could be extended to 140 years, says Richard Miller, a pathologist who does aging research at the University of Michigan.

The Moral Imperative

Furthermore, if rodent experiments are any guide, the future's elderly will be fitter, Miller said, with the average 90-year-old resembling today's 50-year-olds in mind and body.

For these reasons, Miller believes aging research could have a far greater impact on improving public health than trying to cure diseases individually.

The fact that only the rich would have access to life extension technology is not a good enough reason to ban it. . . . Denying treatments to one group of people will not save another.

"If you're really interested in increasing healthy life span, aging research is more likely to get you there in a quick and cost-efficient way than trying to conquer one disease at a time," Miller told LiveScience.

If extending life also prolongs health, as animal studies suggest, then the argument for anti-aging research being a moral imperative is strengthened, says Harris, the University of Manchester bioethicist.

"It is one thing to ask, 'Should we make people immortal?' and answer in the negative. It is quite another to ask whether we should make people immune to heart disease, cancer, dementia, and many other diseases and decide that we should not," Harris contends.

But even if humanity decides to green-light anti-aging research on moral grounds, other thorny ethical issues remain, ethicists say. Uppermost among these is the problem of social injustice.

Who Will Have Access?

Most scientists and ethicists agree that life extension technology will likely be very expensive when first developed, so only a small number of wealthy individuals will be able to afford it. Existing social disparities between rich and poor could become even more pronounced.

The fortunate few who could afford the therapy would not only have significantly longer lives, but more opportunities to amass wealth or political power and to gain control of economic or even cultural institutions, critics say.

Harris points out, however, that the modern world is already rife with similar injustices. The average life expectancy of people in the United States, for example, is about 78 years—but only 34 years in Botswana, which has one of the highest rates of HIV infection in Africa. In Ethiopia, where HIV infection is much less prevalent, life expectancy is 49 years.

Developed nations also have access to medicines and life-saving procedures, such as organ transplants, that are beyond the reach of poor nations. Yet Americans don't typically consider themselves wicked because they have access to things such as kidney transplants while people in other countries don't.

Similarly, Harris says, the fact that only the rich would have access to life extension technology is not a good enough reason to ban it. For one thing, denying treatments to one group of people will not save another. Secondly, new technologies often start off expensive but become cheaper and more widely available with time.

"Injustice may be justifiable in the short term because that is the only way to move to a position where greater justice can be done," Harris told LiveScience. "That's true of all technologies."

People would either have to stop thinking that saving lives is important, or they'll have to stop thinking that there is something wrong with deliberately bringing about death at a certain point.

Centuries of Torment

Another thing to consider is the effect longer lifetimes will have on some of our cherished values, ethicists say. For example, in the United States, the right to life is considered something that every person is entitled to, and both suicide and euthanasia are considered culturally and socially unacceptable.

But in a world where human lives are measured not in decades, but in centuries, or millennia, these values might need to be re-examined. One reason: Immortality will not mean invincibility. Diseases and wars will still kill, strokes will still maim and depression will still be around to blunt the joys of living.

The question of when, if ever, it is OK for people to end their own life or to have someone else end it for them is already a topic of fierce debate. An answer will become even more essential if by telling someone they must live, we condemn them to not just years, but decades or centuries of torment.

Generational Cleansing

Also, Earth can support only so many people. If everyone lived longer, generations would have to be born farther apart to avoid overcrowding.

To ensure ample generational turnover, Harris says, society might need to resort to some kind of "generational cleansing, which would be difficult to justify." This would involve people collectively deciding what length is reasonable for a generation to live and then ensuring individuals died once they reached the end of their term.

Such actions would require radical shifts in our attitudes about suicide and euthanasia, Harris said. People would either have to stop thinking that saving lives is important, or they'll have to stop thinking that there is something wrong with deliberately bringing about death at a certain point.

"We've grown up with a certain set of expectations about life and death, and if those expectations change, a lot of other things will have to change as well," Harris said.

2

Aging Is a Disease That Science Should Cure

Joel Garreau

Joel Garreau is a staff writer for the Washington Post.

Biomedical gerontologist Aubrey de Grey is a larger-than-life character who also has a larger-than-life goal: to cure aging so people can live 1,000 years. Because of his unique personality and the radical nature of his ideas, people often try to write de Grey off as a crackpot, but so far no one has been able to prove that his theories won't work. Other scientists tend to discredit the man rather than his ideas. De Grey reasons that because aging is responsible for two-thirds of all death in the world, then aging itself is a disease that can and should be cured. De Grey approaches aging as though it were an engineering problem that can be systematically solved. He is confident that science and technology will soon allow humans to maintain their bodies over time without further decline, much like classic cars are maintained. De Grey's approach to life extension is bold and revolutionary, but only time will tell if his theories are valid.

Aubrey de Grey may be wrong but, evidence suggests, he's not nuts. This is a no small assertion. De Grey argues that some people alive today will live in a robust and youthful fashion for 1,000 years.

In 2005, an authoritative publication offered $20,000 to any molecular biologist who could demonstrate that de Grey's

Joel Garreau, "The Invincible Man: Aubrey de Grey, 44 Going on 1,000, Wants Out of Old Age," *The Washington Post*, October 31, 2007. http://www.washingtonpost.com. Reprinted with permission.

plan for treating aging as a disease—and curing it—was "so wrong that it was unworthy of learned debate."

Now mere mortals—who may wish to be significantly less mortal—can judge whether de Grey's proposals are "science or fantasy," as the magazine put it. De Grey's much-awaited *Ending Aging: The Rejuvenation Breakthroughs That Could Reverse Human Aging in Our Lifetime* has just been published [2007].

The judges were formidable for that MIT *Technology Review* challenge prize. They included Rodney Brooks, then director of MIT's Computer Science and Artificial Intelligence Laboratory; Nathan Myhrvold, former chief technology officer of Microsoft; and J. Craig Venter, who shares credit for first sequencing the human genome.

With adequate funding, de Grey thinks scientists may, within a decade, triple the remaining life span of late-middle-age mice.

In the end, they decided no scientist had succeeded in blowing de Grey out of the water. "At issue is the conflict between the scientific process and the ambiguous status of ideas that have not yet been subjected to that process," Myhrvold wrote for the judges.

Well yes, that. Plus the question that has tantalized humans forever. What if the only certainty is taxes?

The Mythology of Immortality

Dodging death has long been a dream.

Our earliest recorded legend is that of Gilgamesh, who finds and loses the secret of immortality.

The Greek goddess Eos prevails on Zeus to allow her human lover Tithonus to live eternally, forgetting, unfortunately, to ask that he also not become aged and frail. He winds up such a dried husk she turns him into a grasshopper.

In "It Ain't Necessarily So," [twentieth-century American lyricist] Ira Gershwin writes:

Methus'lah lived nine hundred years
Methus'lah lived nine hundred years
But who calls dat livin' when no gal'll give in
To no man what's nine hundred years.

Aubrey David Nicholas Jasper de Grey, 44, recently of Britain's Cambridge University, advocates not myth but "strategies for engineering negligible senescence," or SENS. It means curing aging.

With adequate funding, de Grey thinks scientists may, within a decade, triple the remaining life span of late-middle-age mice. The day this announcement is made, he believes, the news will hit people like a brick as they realize that their cells could be next. He speculates people will start abandoning risky jobs, such as being police officers, or soldiers.

The real breakthroughs in science are made by serious thinkers who are willing to work on research areas that people think are too controversial or too implausible.

The Man and the Message

De Grey's looks are almost as striking as his ambitions.

His slightly graying chestnut hair is swept back into a ponytail. His russet beard falls to his belly. His mustache—as long as a hand—would have been the envy of Salvador Dali. When he talks about people soon putting a higher premium on health than wealth, he twirls the ends of his mustache back behind his ears, murmuring, "So many women, so much time."

A little over six feet tall and lean—he weighs 147 pounds, the same as in his teenage years—de Grey shows up in a denim work shirt open to the sternum, ripped jeans and scuffed sneakers, looking for all the world like a denizen of Silicon Valley.

Not far from the mark. De Grey's original academic field is computer science and artificial intelligence. He has become the darling of some Silicon Valley entrepreneurs who think changing the world is all in a day's work. Peter Thiel, the co-founder and former CEO of PayPal—who sold it in 2002 for $1.5 billion, pocketing $55 million himself—has dropped $3.5 million on de Grey's Methuselah Foundation.

"I thought he had this rare combination—a serious thinker who had enough courage to break with the crowd," Thiel says. "A lot of people who are not conventional are not serious. But the real breakthroughs in science are made by serious thinkers who are willing to work on research areas that people think are too controversial or too implausible."

At midday in George Washington University's Kogan Plaza off H Street NW, you are surrounded by firm, young flesh. Muscular young men saunter by in sandals, T-shirts and cargo shorts. Young blond women sport clingy, sleeveless tops, over-size sunglasses and the astounding array of subtle variations available in flip-flops and painted toenails.

Is this the future? you ask de Grey.

The Future Is Now

"Yes, it is precisely the future," he says. "Except without people who look as old as you and me."

"Of course the world will be completely different in all manner of ways," de Grey says of the next few decades. His speech is thick, fast and mellifluous [smooth and flowing], with a quality British accent.

"If we want to hit the high points, number one is, there will not be any frail elderly people. Which means we won't be spending all this unbelievable amount of money keeping all those frail elderly people alive for like one extra year the way we do at the moment. That money will be available to spend on important things like, well, obviously, providing the health care to keep us that way, but that won't be anything like so expensive. Secondly, just doing the things we can't afford now, giving people proper education and not just when they're kids, but also proper adult education and retraining and so on.

"Another thing that's going to have to change completely is retirement. For the moment, when you retire, you retire forever. We're sorry for old people because they're going downhill. There will be no real moral or sociological requirement to do that. Sure, there is going to be a need for Social Security as a safety net just as there is now. But retirement will be a periodic thing. You'll be a journalist for 40 years or whatever and then you'll be sick of it and you'll retire on your savings or on a state pension, depending on what the system is. So after 20 years, golf will have lost its novelty value, and you'll want to do something else with your life. You'll get more retraining and education, and go and be a rock star for 40 years, and then retire again and so on."

The mind reels. Will we want to be married to the same person for a thousand years? Will we need religion anymore? Will the planet fill to overflowing?

But first—why are these questions coming up now? And why are we listening to answers from Aubrey de Grey?

Appalled at the Carnage

De Grey became the archenemy of aging in two steps.

"The first stage happened when I was probably 8 or 9 years old. My mother wanted me to practice the piano, and I would resist it.

"She'd already somehow brought me up to be very analytical and introspective. So I realized it was very straightforward. The best possible outcome of my putting in this enormous time at the piano is that I would become a good pianist. That wasn't good enough. I would make a minimal difference in the world, because there were plenty of other very good pianists already. Well, that won't do. What I actually wanted to do with my life is make a difference to the world. That led me into science very quickly."

In his teens he heard the siren song of the the first British microcomputers, the Sinclairs and Acorns, and never looked back. Computer science filled his undergraduate years at Cambridge and became the field in which he spent more than a decade.

The second stage started when he was 26. De Grey fell in love with and married a geneticist, Adelaide Carpenter, who is 19 years his senior.

He learned a lot of biology over the dinner table, he says, and gradually became driven by the notion that "aging is responsible for two-thirds of all death—now that means worldwide 100,000 people every single day—and in the industrialized world, it is something like 90 percent."

The further he got into Carpenter's world and that of her senior colleagues, the more incensed he became that biologists and gerontologists just accept this carnage.

"I was appalled. Utterly appalled. I began to realize the profound difference of motivation and mind-set between scientists on the one hand and technologists and engineers on the other hand."

Pragmatic Thinking

In his world of information technology, the norm is making the world new. Try something and if it doesn't work, try something else. Science doesn't pave the way for engineering, it's the other way around. Intel figures out a way to make wires only a few molecules thick. Why the circuits function is at best of passing interest—as long as they do. Science can take years if not decades to catch up with an adequate explanation of the device's quantum mechanics. It is the final triumph of Edison over Einstein.

The idea of bringing pragmatism to biology made de Grey think "I might be able to make a contribution. I became very aware by this time that biology was critically short of synthe-sizers—people who brought ideas together from disparate fields who came up with new ideas for experimentalists to do." So he got his PhD in biology from Cambridge and started scattering ideas like viruses.

It's just like maintaining the functional life span of a classic car, or a house. . . . The only reason we don't see that in the human body now is that the panel of inter-ventions we have available to us today is not sufficiently comprehensive.

Aging consists of seven critical kinds of damage, according to de Grey. For example, unwholesome goo accumulates in our cells. Our bodies have not evolved means quickly to clean up "intracellular aggregates such as lipofuscin." However, out-side our bodies, microorganisms have eagerly and rapidly evolved to turn this toxic waste into compost. (De Grey made this connection because he knew two things: Lipofuscin is fluorescent and graveyards don't glow in the dark.)

By taking soil samples from an ancient mass grave, de Grey's colleagues in short order found the bacteria that digest lipofuscin as easily as enzymes in our stomachs digest a steak. The trick now is getting those lipofuscin-digesting enzymes into our bodies. That has not yet been done. But, de Grey says, comparable fundamental biotechnology is already in clinical use fighting diseases such as Tay-Sachs. So he sees it as merely an engineering problem.

Examples like this make up the 262 pages at the center of *Ending Aging.*

Repair and Maintenance Are Key

"It's a repair and maintenance approach to extending the functional life span of a human body," de Grey says. "It's just like maintaining the functional life span of a classic car, or a house. We know—because people do it—that there is no limit to how long you can do that. Once you have a sufficiently comprehensive panel of interventions to get rid of damage and maintain these things, then, they can last indefinitely. The only reason we don't see that in the human body now is that the panel of interventions we have available to us today is not sufficiently comprehensive."

All of science rests on ideas that were either unproven hypotheses or crazy speculation at one point.

By 2005, his ideas had attracted enough attention as to no longer be merely controversial. De Grey was being pilloried as a full-blown heretic.

"The idea that a research programme organized around the SENS agenda will not only retard ageing, but also reverse it—creating young people from old ones and do so within our lifetime, is so far from plausible that it commands no respect at all within the informed scientific community," wrote 28 biogerontologists in the journal of the European Molecular Biology Organization. Their recommendation: more of the patient, basic scientific research that is their stock in trade.

"Each idea that we decide to pursue will cost years of work and a great deal of money, so we spend a lot of time—at meetings, seminars and in the library—trying to search for and weigh alternatives, and looking for loopholes in our chain of arguments before they are pointed out to us either by peer reviewers or experimental results.

"Presented by an articulate, witty and colourful proponent, a flashy research agenda might catch the eye of a journalist or meeting organizer who is hunting for attention, publicity and an audience; however, the SENS agenda is easily recognized as a pretence by those with scientific experience.

No One Meets the Challenge

"Why not simply debate with de Grey and let the most convincing arguments win? It is . . . our opinion that pretending that such a collection of ill-founded speculations is a useful topic for debate, let alone a serious guide to research planning, does more harm than good both for science and for society."

The resulting uproar was followed by the put-up-or-shut-up smack-down in MIT *Technology Review*. The upshot was intriguing.

"In our judgment none of the 'refutations' succeeded," Myhrvold, one of the judges, writes in an e-mail.

"It was a bit ironic because they were mostly the work of established scientists in mainstream gerontology who sought to brand de Grey as 'unscientific'—yet the supposed refutations were themselves quite unscientific.

Since the beginning of civilization, we have been aware that aging is ghastly and that aging is utterly inevitable.

"The 'refutations' were either ad hominem attacks on de Grey [attacking the man and not the ideas], or arguments that his ideas would never work (which might be right, but that is what experiments are for), or arguments that portions of de Grey's work rested on other people's ideas. None of these refute the possibility that he is at least partially correct.

"This is *not* to say that the MIT group endorsed de Grey," Myhrvold emphasizes, "or thinks he has proven his case. He hasn't, but admits that upfront. All of science rests on ideas that were either unproven hypotheses or crazy speculations at one point. . . . The sad reality is that most crazy speculations fail. . . . We do not know today how to be forever young for 1,000 years, and I am deeply skeptical that we will figure it out in time for me!"

No Point in Being Miserable

Off the J Street food court at GWU, there is a cafe so metabolically correct that it features not only a vegan service bar, but, separately, a vegetarian service bar, which is not to be confused with the salad bar.

Seems like a good place for lunch with a man intent on immortality.

Not so much.

"I'm getting damn thirsty," de Grey announces.

What appeals to him is the Froggy Bottom Pub on Pennsylvania Avenue. "I like good beer, but I'm not really a snob about beer. I'm perfectly happy to drink Sam Adams, if that's what they have."

Aubrey de Grey is not interested in spending his next centuries miserable. He cheerfully chows down on french fries, heavily crusted deep-fried chicken and two dark beers.

So beyond the question of whether immortality is feasible, is it a good idea? For every Woody Allen who says, "I don't want to achieve immortality through my work; I want to achieve it through not dying," isn't there a Ralph Waldo Emerson who asks, "What would be the use of immortality to a person who cannot use well a half an hour?"

Why is it, when you bring up the idea of living forever—even if robust and healthy, not drooling on your shoes—some people just recoil viscerally?

The "Pro-aging Trance"

"It's probably the majority that recoils viscerally," de Grey says. "It's what I call the pro-aging trance.

"Since the beginning of civilization, we have been aware that aging is ghastly and that aging is utterly inevitable. . . . So we have two choices. Either we spend our lives being preoccupied by this ghastly future or we find some way to get on with our miserably short lives and make the best of it.

"If we do that second thing, which is obviously the right thing to do, then it doesn't matter how irrational that rationalization might be. . . . It could be, well, we're all going to go to heaven. Or it could be, we're going to have overpopulation. Or it could be, it will be boring. Or, dictators will live forever.

"It doesn't matter what the answers are. It's so important for them to maintain their belief that aging is actually not such a bad thing, that they completely suspend any normal rational sense of proportion."

But if people don't die, won't we indeed fill the planet shoulder to shoulder?

"The birthrate is going to have to go down by an order of magnitude," de Grey acknowledges. "But even if that is going to be a severe problem, the question is not, do problems exist? The question is, are they serious enough to outweigh the benefits of saving 100,000 lives a day? That's the fundamental question. If you haven't got an argument that says that it's that serious that we shouldn't save 30 [bleeping] World Trade Centers every [bleeping] day, don't waste my time. It's a sense of proportion thing."

So de Grey soldiers on, not that it is anywhere written that anything he advocates will work. His approach, however, does have echoes in history.

On Oct. 9, 1903, the *New York Times* wrote:

"The flying machine which will really fly might be evolved by the combined and continuous efforts of mathematicians and mechanicians in from one million to ten million years."

On the same day, on Kill Devil Hill, N.C., in his diary, a bicycle mechanic named Orville Wright wrote:

"We unpacked rest of goods for new machine."

3

Life Extension Raises Complex Social Issues

George Dvorsky

George Dvorsky is the president of the Toronto Transhumanist Association, a nonprofit organization devoted to encouraging the use of technology to transcend the limitations of the human body.

Most arguments promoting life extension focus on the idea that life is intrinsically valuable at any age. Life extensionists, quite simply, believe that life is good and death is bad. They are acutely aware that people die every day from age-related diseases, and they want to change that. However, little has been written about the social and economic benefits that radical life extension would bring. For example, because people would live so much longer, it would give them a greater personal stake in the future and would lead to more sustainable public polices in many areas. Such positive benefits of life extension are just starting to gain recognition and support as they are used to refute the arguments of those who oppose the development and use of such technologies. Radical life extension is an unavoidable eventuality modern scientific progress. The dialog must begin now about its potential benefits and how to manage increased human longevity in the long term.

George Dvorsky, Transcription of George Dvorsky's and Anders Sandberg's talks from the IEET's July 23rd Longevity Dividend Seminar: Popular Arguments For and Against Longevity, IEET, July 23, 2007. http://www.sentientdevelopments.com. Reproduced by permission.

To date, the arguments for . . . radical life extension have been almost exclusively about why life is valuable, not really having the evidence from a social or economic perspective why life extension is viable. One can make the case that arguments for the social good of life extension are beginning to coalesce. I find that arguments for life extension tend to be somewhat on the offensive. We are under attack, and many of the arguments are meant to deflect criticism.

There are four broad categories to the arguments of pro-longevists: the value of life and undesirability of death, the ethical and legal right to life extension, that there are desirable social consequences, and that it is more a matter of working toward the inevitable than striving toward the feasible.

Life extensionists are cognizant of the fact that people are dying every day of age-related diseases.

Life is good, death is bad. That pretty much says it all for life extensionists. There is the general notion that death at 17 is tragic, while death at 87 is natural. That is based on our conditioned response and expectations regarding maximum lifespan. If we could live to 1000, we would consider the death of someone at 350 to be just as tragic. The Greek philosopher Epicurus stated that death is nothing to us when we are dead. That said, death is most certainly to the frustration of the living. People who desire to go on living, they have objectives for the future, objectives which they hope to translate into real experiences, and death might be seen as the denier of future experience. A great quote from J.R.R. Tolkien, "There is no such thing as a natural death. Nothing that happens to Man is ever natural, since his presence calls the whole world into question. All men must die, but for every man his death is an accident. And even if he knows it and consents to it, an unjustifiable violation." The quote is the obverse to [bioethicist]

Leon Kass's assertion that the finitude of human life is a blessing for every individual, whether he knows it or not.

Another argument is that death is wasteful, destroying memories and experiences. Moreover, it is a terrible thing to have to deal with death. Eliezer Yudkowsky, who experienced the death of his sibling a few years ago, wrote that "No sentient being deserves such a thing." Life extensionists are cognizant of the fact that people are dying every day of age-related diseases.

With longer life expectancy, people will have a personal stake in the future. And this will lead to more sustainable policy.

Ethical and Legal Issues

Let me skim the ethical and legal issues underlying the argument for life extension. Some might define the ability to transform and manipulate our bodies as we see fit as being an issue of civil liberties, personal freedom and choice. In denying affluent groups the right to life extension out of consideration for the societal divides, John Davis has said that in other contexts taking from the haves is only justifiable when it makes the have-nots more than marginally better off. The IEET [Institute for Ethics and Emerging Technologies] is working to ensure that these technologies have as broad access as possible.

As for the desirable social consequences, it has been said that it would result in an increased concern for personal responsibility. Individuals would have a longer time to deal with the repercussions of their negative actions. Given longer lifespans, people could cultivate deeper and more profound wisdom. Nick Bostrom has argued that with longer life expectancy, people will have a personal stake in the future. And this will lead to more sustainable policy. It also makes utilitarians happy. Michael Anissimov has said that life extension is important to utilitarians because billions of people want it.

Another interesting take, one I am somewhat partial to, is that in opposing life extension we're actually talking about arguing against the [flow]. This argument says that life extension at some point is inevitable given the accelerating rate of technological progress and the human desire to exist. We should therefore be talking about how to manage the process of increasing longevity. It has been argued that life extension is the logical extension of the medical sciences. Another way of looking at it, instead of arguing for the abolition of death, one might argue for the medical conquest of disease up to and including age-related illness.

Injunctions against life extension once it exists would open up a Pandora's box of problems. The demand for illegal life extension technologies would have to be endorsed by a transglobal regulatory agency, foreseeably leading to the proliferation of black markets and the possibility for risky end-user experimentation.

Is It Feasible?

Finally there is the issue of feasibility. If we can show that the seemingly practical inhibitors to life extension are surmountable, non-tractable problems, in what ways are we now obligated to do these things? Aubrey de Grey has argued that we are responsible for future generations. Technology experts point out that many opponents to life extension ignore the progress being made in remediations to reduce our global footprint, harness safe alternative high-energy sources, and so on. Quoting Ray Kurzweil, "We need to expand our intelligence and our capacity for experience, which is exactly what new technologies will enable us to do."

4

Early Intervention Extends Life and Ensures Health

S. Jay Olshansky, Daniel Perry, Richard A. Miller, and Robert N. Butler

S. Jay Olshansky is professor of epidemiology and biostatistics at the University of Illinois in Chicago. Daniel Perry is executive director for the Alliance for Aging Research in Washington, D.C. Richard A. Miller is professor of pathology at the University of Michigan, Ann Arbor. Robert N. Butler is president and CEO of the International Longevity Center in New York.

Medical science now understands that aging plays a major role in the diseases from which modern humans die, such as cancer and heart disease. It is also now clear that the aging process can be slowed or delayed with the right medical interventions. Offering such anti-aging treatments not only would save and extend lives, it would keep people healthy longer and thereby create economic wealth. How quickly this becomes a reality depends on public policy and financial support for anti-aging research. The government should significantly increase funding for the study of the biology of aging. That way, science can better understand how aging predisposes humans to diseases later in life and can work to find treatments for aging itself. Slowing down the aging process means extending healthy life. If medical science is able to work toward this goal now, the next generation will be able to reap the benefits.

S. Jay Olshansky, Daniel Perry, Richard A. Miller, and Robert N. Butler, "In Pursuit of the Longevity Dividend: What Should We Be Doing to Prepare for the Unprecedented Aging of Humanity?" *The Scientist*, March 2006, pp. 28–35. © 2006 *The Scientist*. Republished with permission of The Scientist.

Imagine an intervention, such as a pill, that could signifi- cantly reduce your risk of cancer. Imagine an intervention that could reduce your risk of stroke, or dementia, or arthri- tis. Now, imagine an intervention that does all these things, and at the same time reduces your risk of everything else un- desirable about growing older: including heart disease, diabe- tes, Alzheimer and Parkinson disease, hip fractures, osteoporo- sis, sensory impairments, and sexual dysfunction. Such a pill may sound like fantasy, but aging interventions already do this in animal models. And many scientists believe that such an intervention is a realistically achievable goal for people. People already place a high value on both quality and length of life, which is why children are immunized against infectious dis- eases. In the same spirit, we suggest that a concerted effort to slow aging begin immediately—because it will save and ex- tend lives, improve health, and create wealth.

The experience of aging is about to change. Humans are approaching old age in unprecedented numbers, and this gen- eration and all that follow have the potential to live longer, healthier lives than any in history. These changing demo- graphics also carry the prospect of overwhelming increases in age-related disease, frailty, disability, and all the associated costs and social burdens. The choices we make now will have a profound influence on the health and the wealth of current and future generations.

Gerontology Comes of Age

Gerontology has grown beyond its historical and traditional image of disease management and palliative care for the old, to the scientific study of aging processes in humans and in other species—the latter is known as biogerontology. In recent decades biogerontologists have gained significant insight into the causes of aging. They've revolutionized our understanding of the biology of life and death. They've dispelled long-held misconceptions about aging and its effects, and offered for the first time a real scientific foundation for the feasibility of extending and improving life.

The belief that aging is an immutable process, programmed by evolution, is now known to be wrong.

The idea that age-related illnesses are independently influenced by genes and/or behavioral risk factors has been dispelled by evidence that genetic and dietary interventions can retard nearly all late-life diseases in parallel. Several lines of evidence in models ranging from simple eukaryotes to mammals suggest that our own bodies may well have "switches" that influence how quickly we age. These switches are not set in stone; they are potentially adjustable.

Biogerontologists have progressed far beyond merely describing cellular aging, cell death, free radicals, and telomere shortening, to actually manipulating molecular machinery and cell functions.(1) These recent scientific breakthroughs have nothing in common with the claims of entrepreneurs selling alleged anti-aging interventions they say can slow, stop, or reverse human aging (see "Your money for your life" on pg. 33 for a peek at this industry). No such treatment yet exists.

Nevertheless, the belief that aging is an immutable process, programmed by evolution, is now known to be wrong. In recent decades, our knowledge of how, why, and when aging processes take place has progressed so much that many scientists now believe that this line of research, if sufficently promoted, could benefit people alive today.(2)(3) Indeed, the science of aging has the potential to do what no drug, surgical procedure, or behavior modification can do—extend our years of youthful vigor and simultaneously postpone all the costly, disabling, and lethal conditions expressed at later ages.

In addition to the obvious health benefits, enormous economic benefits would accrue from the extension of healthy life. By extending the time in the lifespan when higher levels of physical and mental capacity are expressed, people would remain in the labor force longer, personal income and savings would increase, age-entitlement programs would face less pressure from shifting demographics, and there is reason to believe that national economies would flourish. The science of aging has the potential to produce what we refer to as a "Longevity Dividend" in the form of social, economic, and health bonuses both for individuals and entire populations—a dividend that would begin with generations currently alive and continue for all that follow.

The underlying biological changes that predispose every-one to fatal and disabling diseases and disorders are caused by the processes of aging. It therefore stands to reason that an intervention that delays aging should be-come one of our highest priorities.

We contend that conditions are ripe today for the aggressive pursuit of the Longevity Dividend by seeking the technical means to intervene in the biological processes of aging in our species, and by ensuring that the resulting interventions become widely available.

Why Act Now?

Consider what is likely to happen if we don't. Take, for instance, the impact of just one age-related disorder, Alzheimer disease (AD). For no other reason than the inevitable shifting demographics, the number of Americans stricken with AD will rise from 4 million today to as many as 16 million by midcentury.(4) This means that more people in the United States will have AD by 2050 than the entire current population of the Netherlands. Globally, AD prevalence is expected to rise to 45 million by 2050, with three of every four patients with AD living in a developing nation.(5) The US economic toll is currently $80–$100 billion, but by 2050 more than $1 trillion will be spent annually on AD and related dementias. The impact of this single disease will be catastrophic, and this is just one example.

Cardiovascular disease, diabetes, cancer, and other age-related problems account for billions of dollars siphoned away for "sick care." Imagine the problems in many developing nations where there is little or no formal training in geriatric health care. For instance, in China and India the elderly will outnumber the total current US population by midcentury. The demographic wave is a global phenomenon that appears to be leading health care financing into an abyss.

Nations may be tempted to continue attacking diseases and disabilities of old age separately, as if they were unrelated to one another. This is the way most medicine is practiced and medical research is conducted today. The National Institutes of Health in the United States are organized under the premise that specific diseases and disorders be attacked individually. More than half of the National Institute on Aging budget in the United States is devoted to AD. But the underlying biological changes that predispose everyone to fatal and disabling diseases and disorders are caused by the processes of aging.(6) It therefore stands to reason that an intervention that delays aging should become one of our highest priorities.

If we succeed in slowing aging by seven years, the age-specific risk of death, frailty, and disability will be reduced by approximately half at every age.

Health and Longevity Create Wealth

According to studies undertaken at the International Longevity Center and at universities around the world, the extension of healthy life creates wealth for individuals and the nations in which they live.(7) Healthy older individuals accumulate more savings and investments than those beset by illness. They tend to remain productively engaged in society. They spark economic booms in so-called mature markets, including financial services, travel, hospitality, and intergenerational transfers to younger generations. Improved health status also leads to less absenteeism from school and work and is associated with better education and higher income.

A successful intervention that delays aging would do more than yield a one-time benefit, after which, one might argue, the same exorbitant health-care expenses would ensue. Life extension already achieved among animals suggests that delayed aging may produce a genuine compression of mortality and morbidity.(8) Calorie-restricted animals not only experience a reduction in their risk of death, but also experience declines in the risk of a wide variety of age-sensitive, nonlethal conditions such as cataracts, kidney diseases, arthritis, cognitive decline, collagen cross linking, immune senescence, and many others.(9) If this could be achieved in people, the benefits to health and vitality would begin immediately and continue throughout the remainder of the lifespan. Thus the costly period of frailty and disability would be experienced during a shorter duration of time before death. This compression of mortality and morbidity would create financial gains not only because aging populations will have more years to contribute, but also because there will be more years during which age-entitlement and healthcare programs are not used.

A Maturing Science

Centuries ago, the French naturalist Buffon observed that aging exhibits common characteristics across species. Recent work in genetics and in the comparative biology of aging confirms these impressions and provides important clues about how to develop effective interventions that delay aging. It is now clear that some of the hormones and cellular pathways that influence the rate of aging in lower organisms also contribute to many of the manifestations of aging that we see in humans, such as cancers, cararacts, heart disease, arthritis, and cognitive decline. These manifestations occur in much the same way in other animals and for the same biological reasons.(10) (For more on one example see "Aging research for the dogs"). Several experiments have demonstrated that by manipulating certain genes, altering reproduction, reducing caloric intake, and changing the signal pathways of specific physiological mechanisms, the duration of life of both inverte-brates and mammals can be extended.(11)(12) Some of the genes involved, such as *PIT1*, *PROP1*, and *GHR/BP*, modulate the levels of hormones that affect growth and maturation; others, such as *p66SHC*, help individual cells avoid injury and death. No one is suggesting that alteration of these genes in human would be practical, useful, or ethical, but it does seem likely that further investigation may yield important clues about intervening pharmacologically.

Genes that slow growth in early life—such as those that produce differences between large, middle-size, and miniature dogs—typically postpone all the signs and symptoms of aging in parallel. A similar set of hormonal signals, related in se-quence and action to human insulin, insulin-like growth fac-tor (IGF-I), or both, are involved in aging, life span, and pro-tection against injury in worms, flies, and mice, and extend life span in all of those animals. These hormones help indi-vidual cells buffer the toxic effects of free radicals, radiation damage, environmental toxins, and protein aggregates that contribute to various late-life malfunctions.

An extension of disease-free lifespan of approximately 40% has already been achieved repeatedly in experiments with mice and rats.(13-16) These examples, provide powerful new systems to study how aging processes influence disease expres-sion and will yield clues about where to look for interventions that can slow aging in people in a safe and effective way. Since many of the biological pathways of aging are conserved also in simple invertebrate species such as fruit flies, it should be possible to experimentally evaluate candidate intervention strategies rapidly.

Some people, including a proportion of centenarians, live most of their lives free from frailty and disability. Genetics plays a critical role in their healthy survival. Identifying variation in these subgroups of humans holds great potential for improving public health. For example, microsomal transfer protein (MTP) on chromosome 4 has been identified as a longevity modifier in a sample of centenarians(17); there is strong evidence linking a common variant of *KLOTHO*, the KL-VS allele, to human longevity(18); and it has been demonstrated that lipoprotein particle sizes promote a healthy aging phenotype through codon 405 valine variation in cholesteryl ester transfer protein (*CETP*).(19)

Given the speed at which the study of aging has advanced and the ability to obtain research results quickly from the study of short-lived species, scientists have reason to be confident that a Longevity Dividend is a plausible outcome of aging research.

The Target

What we have in mind is not the unrealistic pursuit of dramatic increases in life expectancy, let alone the kind of biological immorality best left to science fiction novels.(20) Rather, we envision a goal that is realistically achievable: a modest deceleration in the rate of aging sufficient to delay all aging-related diseases and disorders by about seven years.(21) This target was chosen because the risk of death and most other negative attributes of aging tends to rise exponentially throughout the adult lifespan with a doubling time of approximately seven years.(22) Such a delay would yield health and longevity benefits greater than what would be achieved with the elimination of cancer or heart disease.(23) And we believe it can be achieved for generations now alive.

If we succeed in slowing aging by seven years, the age-specific risk of death, frailty, and disability will be reduced by approximately half at every age. People who reach the age of 50 in the future would have the health profile and disease risk of today's 43-year-old; those aged 60 would resemble current 53-year-olds, and so on. Equally important, once achieved, this seven-year delay would yield equal health and longevity benefits for all subsequent generations, much the same way children born in most nations today benefit from the discovery and development of immunizations.

A growing chorus of scientists agrees that this objective is scientifically and technologically feasible.(24) How quickly we see success depends in part on the priority and support devoted to the effort. Certainly such a great goal—to win back, on average, seven years of healthy life—requires and deserves significant resources in time, talent, and treasury. But with the mammoth investment already committed in caring for the sick as they age, and the pursuit of ever-more-expensive treatments and surgical procedures for existing fatal and disabling diseases, the pursuit of the Longevity Dividend would be modest by comparison. In fact, because a healthier, longer-lived population will add significant wealth to the economy, an investment in the Longevity Dividend would likely pay for itself.

A successful effort to extend healthy life by slowing aging may very well be one of the most important gifts that our generation can give.

The Recommendation

The NIH is funded at $28 billion in 2006, but less than 0.1% of that amount goes to understanding the biology of aging and how it predisposes us to a suite of costly diseases and disorders expressed at later ages. We are calling on Congress to invest $3 billion annually to this effort, or about 1% of the current Medicare budget of $309 billion, and to provide the organizational and intellectual infrastructure and other related resources to make this work.

Specifically, we recommend that one-third of this budget ($1 billion) be devoted to the basic biology of aging with a focus on genomics and regenerative medicine as they relate to longevity science. Another third should be devoted to age-related diseases as part of a coordinated trans-NIH effort. One-sixth ($500 million) should be devoted to clinical trials with proportionate representation of older persons (aged 65+) that include head-to-head studies of drugs or interventions including lifestyle comparisons, cost-effectiveness studies, and the development of a national system for postmarketing surveillance.

The remaining $500 million should go to a national preventive medicine research initiative that would include studies of safety and health in the home and workplace and address issues of physical inactivity and obesity as well as genetic and other early-life pathological influences. This last category would include studies of the social and economic means to effect positive changes in health behaviors in the face of current health crises—obesity and diabetes—that can lower life expectancy. Elements of the budget could be phased in over time, and it would be appropriate to use funds within each category for research training and the development of appropriate infrastructure. We also strongly encourage the development of an international consortium devoted to this task, as all nations would benefit from securing the Longevity Dividend.

With this effort, we believe it will be possible to intervene in aging among the baby boom cohorts, and all generations after them would enjoy the health and economic benefits of delayed aging. Such a monetary commitment would be small when compared to that spent each year on Medicare alone, but it would pay dividends an order of magnitude greater than the investment. And it would do so for current and future generations.

In our view, the scientific evidence strongly supports the idea that the time has arrived to invest in the future of humanity by encouraging the commensurate political will, public support, and resources required to slow aging, and to do so now so that most people currently alive might benefit from the investment. A successful effort to extend healthy life by slowing aging may very well be one of the most important gifts that our generation can give.

References

1. H. Warner, "Twenty years of progress in biogerontology," National Institute on Aging, 2005.

2. R.M. Miller, "Extending life: Scientific prospects and political obstacles," *Milbank Q*, 80:155–74, 2002.

3. Public Agenda, "The science of aging gracefully: Scientists and the public talk about aging research," The Alliance for Aging Research and the American Federation for Aging research, 2005.

4. F. Liesi et al., "Alzheimer disease in the US population: Prevalence estimates using the 2000 census,"*Arch Neurol*, 60:1119–22, 2003.

5. Alzheimer's Disease Annual Report, Alzheimer's Disease International, 2004–2005; www.frost.com/prod/servlet/dsd-fact-file.pag?docid=38565311.

6. R.N. Butler et al., "The aging factor in health and disease: The promise of basic research on aging, Special Report, *Aging Clin Exp Res*, 16:104–12,

7. D. Bloom, D. Canning, "The health and wealth of nations," *Science*, 287:1207–9, 2000.

8. M. Vergara et al., "Hormone-treated Snell dwarf mice regain fertitlity but remain long-lived and disease resistant," *J Gerontol A Biol Sci Med Sci*, 59:1244–50, 2004.

9. R.A. Miller, S.N. Austad, "Growth and aging: Why do big dogs die young?" in *Handbook of the Biology of Aging*, E.J. Masoro, S.N. Austad, eds., New York: Academic press, 2006, pp. 512–33.

10. D. Sinclair, L. Guarente, "Unlocking the secrets of longevity genes," *Sci Am*, March 2006, [in press].

11. M. Tatar et al., "The endocrine regulation of aging by insulin-like signals," *Science*, 299:1346–51, 2003.

12. R. Weindruch, R.S. Sohal, "Seminars in medicine of the Beth Israel Deaconess Medical Center. Caloric intake and aging," *New Engl J Med*, 337:986–94, 1997.

13. H.M. Brown-Borg et al., "Dwarf mice and the aging process," *Nature*, 384:33, 1996.

14. K. Flurkey et al., "Lifespan extension and delayed immune and collagen aging in mutant mice with defects in growth hormone production," *Proc Natl Acad Sci*, 98:6736–41, 2001.

15. B.P. Yu et al., "Nutritional influences on aging of Fischer 344 rats: I. Physical, metabolic, and longevity characteristics," *J Gerontol*, 40:657–70, 1985.

16. R. Weindruch, R.I. Walford, *The Retardatiion of Aging and Disease by Dietary Restriction*, Springfield, Ill., Charles C. Thomas, 1988.

17. B.J. Geesaman et al., "Haplotype-based identification of a microsomal transfer protein marker associated with the human lifespan," *Proc Natl Acad Sci*, 100:14115–20, 2003.

18. D.E. Arking et al., "Association between a functional variant of the *KLOTHO* gene and high-density lipoprotein cholesterol, blood pressure, stroke, and longevity," *Circ Res*, 96:412, 2005.

19. N. Barzilai et al., "Unique lipoprotein phenotype and genotype associated with exceptional longevity," *JAMA*, 290:2030–40, 2003.

20. H. Warner et al., "Science fact and the SENS agenda," *EMBO Reports*, 6:1006–8, 2005.

21. S.J. Olshansky, "Can we justify efforts to slow the rate of aging in humans?" Presentation before the annual meeting of the Gerontological Society of America, 2003.

22. R.N. Butler, J.A. Brody, eds., *Delaying the Onset of Late-life Dysfunction*, New York: Springer Publishing, 1995.

23. S.J. Olshansky, "Simultaneous/multiple cause delay: An epidemiological approach to projecting mortality," *J Gerontol*, 42:358–65, 1987.

24. S.J. Olshansky et al., "Position statement on human aging," *J Gerontol Biol Sci*, 57a: B1–B6, 2002.

5

Longer Lifespans Could Make People Feel Dissatisfied and Less Human

Ker Than

Ker Than is a staff writer for LiveScience, a science-oriented Internet content provider.

Radically extending the human lifespan could have serious consequences for how humans perceive themselves. Aging is not a disease, but rather a process that helps people make sense of their lives. Death is a necessary part of living. If humans do not grow old and die, the rhythm of natural life is disturbed and it alters the very definition of what it means to be human. Because life is finite, it can be perceived as more special. Another perspective on this issue is that if aging is eliminated and the lifespan greatly extended, boredom and prolonged unhappiness may also become critical issues for some people, which could lead to an increase in suicide.

In Oscar Wilde's novel, "The Picture of Dorian Gray," the main character barters his soul for eternal youth but becomes wicked and immoral in the process.

Leon Kass believes humanity risks striking a similar Faustian bargain if it pursues technology that extends life spans beyond what is natural.

If our species ever does unlock the secrets of aging and learns to live forever, we might not lose our souls, but, like

Dorian, we will no longer be human either, says Kass, a bioethicist at the University of Chicago and a longtime critic of life extension research. For Kass, to argue that life is better without death is to argue "that human life would be better being something other than human."

Kass' position is controversial, but it gets at some of the central issues surrounding the life extension debate: What is aging? Is it a disease to be cured or a natural part of life? If natural, is it necessarily good for us?

Virtues of Mortality

In numerous presentations and papers throughout the years, Kass has argued for what he calls the "virtues of mortality." First among them is the effect mortality has on our interest in and engagement with life. To number our days, Kass contends, "is the condition for making them count and for treasuring and appreciating all that life brings."

Kass also believes that the process of aging itself is important because it helps us make sense of our lives.

I don't think one can make our humanity dependent on the length of our life. . . . Even if we live to be 500, we'll still be human beings.

A 2003 staff working paper drawn up by the U.S. President's Council of Bioethics—then headed by Kass—states: "The very experience of spending a life, and of becoming *spent* in doing so, contributes to our sense of accomplishment and commitment, and to our sense of the meaningfulness of the passage of time, and of our passage through it."

Technology that retards aging, the report argues, would "sever age from the moorings of nature, time and maturity."

Reality Sets In

Daniel Callahan of the Hastings Center, a bioethics research institute in New York, agrees that the pursuit of extension technology is unwise, but thinks Kass' views are too extreme.

"His view is that the fact that we're going to die makes us think more seriously about our life," Callahan said. "I don't know if that's necessarily true. I'm 75 now, and that certainly hasn't been my experience."

Callahan also questions the idea that our humanity is somehow tied to our sense of finitude.

"I don't think one can make our humanity dependent on the length of our life," Callahan told LiveScience. "Even if we live to be 500, we'll still be human beings."

Besides, other critics say, Kass is primarily concerned with immortality, something that most scientists say will never happen. "There is no research into extending the life span thousands of years," said Richard Miller, a pathologist at the University of Michigan. "That's fantasy."

Even when applied to the more modest and realistic goal of extending our life spans by a few years or decades, or even doubling it, Kass' arguments don't hold up, said Chris Hackler, head of the Division of Medical Humanities at the University of Arkansas.

Longer life means more time for boredom to creep in.

"We live [longer now] than we did a century ago, but that doesn't mean we take life any less seriously or less creatively, so I don't know why projecting that for a doubled lifespan would be radically different," Hackler said in a recent telephone interview.

Hackler also points out that even if people could potentially live to be 180, they could still die from accidents or disease: It is not the knowledge that we will die by some certain age that spurs us to make the most of life, Hackler says, but the awareness that we can die at any moment—and that will not change even if we are immortal.

Eternal Bore

Instead of worrying about what longer life will do to our sense of humanity, Callahan and Hackler wonder what the heck people are going to do with all their extra time. Longer life means more time for boredom to creep in.

"Let's face it, most people's jobs aren't all that fascinating," Hackler said. "They put in a 9-to-5 and they're glad to have the weekend. So you wonder if having twice as much of this is a good thing, or if you'd get totally burned out."

Hackler can't imagine himself ever getting tired of living, but he knows not everyone will feel same way. Determining how much ennui [boredom] the average person can bear will be important if life extension ever becomes a reality, Hackler says, because extended boredom could result in prolonged unhappiness or higher incidences of suicide.

Against concerns of chronic boredom, those in favor of extending life spans significantly say, "speak for yourself." Aubrey de Grey from the University of Cambridge believes longer life will invigorate people to do the things they've always wanted to do. "There are things that no one attempts today because they feel they'll never get them done in a lifetime," de Grey writes. "If a lifetime is a lot longer they'll try them."

Callahan thinks this kind of thinking gives the average person too much credit.

"I don't believe that if you give most people longer lives, even in better health, they are going to find new opportunities and new initiatives," Callahan has said. "They will want to come and play more golf maybe, but they aren't going to contribute lots of brand new ideas, at least the ones I know."

Even if people had all the time in the world, they will never be able to do *all* the things they wanted to do, Callahan argues.

"Even if you've seen everything, you might say 'Well, I want to go see India once again,'" he told LiveScience. "It seems there's a possibly never-ending cycle there."

If people end up doing *most* of the things on their to-do lists by the time they reach 80, then perhaps that is good enough.

"The fact that there are still some countries that I've never been to does not ruin my life," Callahan said. "I've never been to Nepal or Antarctica but it's hard to work that up to some great tragedy of my life."

6

Opposition to Life Extension Is Based on Myths

João Pedro de Magalhães

João Pedro de Magalhães is a Belgium-based futurist and micro-biologist who specializes in aging issues.

Most people who object to extending the human lifespan by curing aging base their objections on myths and misinformation. Aging is neither inevitable nor universal, and it is not necessarily true that a shorter life is more precious. Modern science will make it possible to extend good health as well as life. Although not everyone in the world will be able to benefit equally from anti-aging technologies, these disparities are not sufficient reason to withhold their development and use. Populations that live longer would be economically profitable because people would work more years and remain healthier longer than they now do. Curing aging would reshape society, but there is no reason to think that would be a negative thing. Overpopulation remains a serious consideration but it is one that can be thoughtfully addressed.

Aging fosters sickness and disability, increases human suffering, and makes us more likely to die. Yet there are a number of possible objections to the endeavor of curing aging. Most of these are unfounded myths and hence easy to disprove. This essay draws on my own lectures on the subject and attempts to answer the most commonly raised questions and concerns about a possible cure for aging and the work of gerontologists.

João Pedro de Magalhães, "Should We Cure Aging?" Senescence.info, 2004. http://www.senescence.info. Reproduced by permission.

Myth #1: Aging Is Natural and So We Shouldn't Fight It

First of all, and contrary to popular belief, aging is not universal. A number of complex species, such as lobsters, rockfishes, and tortoises, do not show signs of aging. Therefore, aging is not a prerequisite to life. Aging is neither inevitable nor universal.

We aim not just to make elderly people live longer but—by improving the health—diminish, not extend, their suffering.

Secondly, humankind is, in a sense, a struggle against nature. We have antibiotics and vaccines because we don't want to be sick, which would be the *natural* outcome in most cases. Yes, some people who drive cars, take medicines, wear glasses, receive e-mail, watch television, and don't have to kill their own dinner think life-extension is unnatural. I just think that life-extension is another adaptation of humans and one that, like many others, will make us live longer, healthier, and happier lives.

Myth #2: What's the Point of Extending Life if We Are Old?

This is a common misconception about research on the biology of aging. The ultimate goal of my work and that of many biogerontologists is to preserve and extend health, well-being, and life, not age-related debilitation. We aim not just to make elderly people live longer but—by improving their health—diminish, not extend, their suffering. What we want is to find ways to extend healthy lifespan by postponing disease and eventually eradicate all forms of age-related involution. In other words, to find a cure for aging, an intervention that permits us to avoid aging and all pathologies associated with it.

More than improving the quality of life of the elderly, we want to avoid having elderly patients in the first place.

According to my calculations, if we were to cure aging that would result in an average longevity of at least 1,200 years in industrial countries. This assumes one would be forever young in body and mind. People would still die from accidents, infectious diseases, etc. After all, children and teenagers die too even though they are not yet aged.

Myth #3: A Finite Lifespan Is Best Enjoyed

The ancient Greeks had an average longevity of 19 years and I'm pretty sure we are happier than them. In fact, longevity increased 50% over the past century and even so quality of life has clearly increased. Entertainment evolves and social adjustments occur. A cure for aging would not mean an eternal life, for one could still die. It would mean an average lifespan of 1,200 years, but life would still be finite. In addition, people would always have a choice to end their lives. At present we don't have a choice of living past 122 years, which is the longest anyone has ever lived so far. With a cure for aging each of us would have a choice to live 100, 200, 1,000 or even more years.

Curing aging and extending healthy lifespan would be profitable for nations.

Myth #4: Why Should Death Be Better Than Life?

This is actually an interesting philosophical question. Many societies, including Western societies, value death in some circumstances—e.g., death in combat, death to save other lives, etc. Other societies are even more extreme and you can always argue that I don't know what is it like to be dead. As an atheist, I clearly favour life to death. It's true I won't feel death.

But if I compare death to its opposite, I always choose life. For those who disagree suicide is always a solution.

Myth #5: Not Everyone Would Benefit from a Cure for Aging

The issue of justice is commonly raised when discussing life-extension. Of course it is impossible to predict the price a fictitious cure for aging would have. Yet a number of medical breakthroughs are not immediately available to everyone. The early antibiotics were available only to an elite and a number of present technologies, such as CAT scans or heart transplants, are not available to everyone. That is not a reason for us to ban pacemakers or regenerative medicine. We don't deny heart transplants just because they're not accessible to everyone. We can't deny health and life just because some people lack healthcare. Besides, even if curing aging is initially expensive, with mass production and widespread facilities one can expect it to be available to everyone, at least in industrialized nations.

When Vasco da Gama and Christopher Columbus explored the world they left death and injustice on the shores of Europe. Neil Armstrong walked on the moon without world peace and Tim Berners-Lee didn't wait for an end of poverty to invent the Internet. Yet all the discoveries and endeavors of these men benefited their societies and humankind in general. There are no ideal circumstances. Setting new limits and making new discoveries eventually improves the lives of everyone.

Myth #6: Economic Disaster Would Result with the Collapse of Health Care

No, of course not. In fact, curing aging and extending healthy lifespan would be profitable for nations. The economic value of increased longevity is estimated at $2.4 trillion per year for the US alone. The greatest burden on healthcare comes from the elderly and the trend is for expenses with old age to increase as the percentage of people over 65 years old rises worldwide. If aging is not tackled, societies in the 21st century will consist of a large proportion of frail, elderly people, which will result in a serious financial burden. Therefore, curing aging would be economically sound. People would live longer but also work longer and thus be more productive. Without the declining years of old age, healthcare and the economy would benefit from a cure for aging. . . .

Myth #7: Overpopulation Would Be a Problem

When talking about life-extension it is intuitive we consider overpopulation as a possible problem. In the 1970s there was a current of thought known as the *Malthusianism* that predicted major problems due to overpopulation by the year 2000. These predictions failed miserably because their proponents did not take into account technological progress made in agriculture, etc. Therefore, we cannot see breakthroughs in aging research as isolated events but rather consider these in the overall evolution of the social organism. The world's population increased almost four-fold in the past century and yet today we have a life quality unparalleled in human history. In fact, population growth with a cure for aging should still be slower than during the "baby boom."

Overpopulation in some regions of the world, such as southeast Asia, may be aggravated by a cure for aging. Yet letting people die to control overpopulation is morally repugnant. If we cure aging and overpopulation becomes a problem in some regions, then we must find other solutions besides letting people die.

Myth #8: Human Trials Would Be Dangerous

This problem occurs with any other medical breakthrough. Following animal tests, human trials begin in a few people.

Only after the security and quality of the product being tested is assured can the company commercialize it. Certain products can escape these regulations using a variety of legal stratagems, but that is a general problem in the biomedical industry, not specific of anti-aging research.

Even if we cure aging, individuals will still be able to choose whether they wanted to age or not.

Myth #9: Humankind as We Know It Would Change

Certainly, but that is not necessarily a "bad thing." Humankind changed considerably since the Roman Empire and yet those changes now allow us to live longer, happier lives. A cure for aging would reshape society but nothing suggests such changes would be negative to humankind. People do not exist to serve society. Society exists to serve people, to make people happier and fight solitude. In the same way the world is a better place to live in due to the many changes that occurred in the past centuries, a cure for aging would make it an even better place thanks to the decrease in suffering and the increase in health. Although no one can foresee the long-term consequences of a cure for aging, and there are potential problems such as intergenerational differences in wealth and status, society could profit. And people would certainly profit.

Myth #10: We Should Have Other Priorities on Earth

Of course there are many problems and injustices in our world. Many nations face hunger, poverty, and widespread disease. Yet, as mentioned in regard to the justice issue on myth #5, this does not mean industrialized nations must abandon expensive medicines. Besides, the technology to solve poor countries' problems is already here—i.e., sustainable agriculture, vaccines, birth control, etc.—and it is up to these nations to implement them.

Aging is the major problem we face in our society. It is or will be the major cause of suffering and pain for me and the ones I love. This holds true for industrialized nations and Western civilization and that is why aging must be a top priority.

Myth #11: Overall, Curing Aging Is Ethically Wrong

Not so. According to the principles of bioethics, like the principle of beneficence, since curing aging would benefit people, not harm them, it is not ethically wrong. Anti-aging therapies would serve to the amelioration of the many diseases for which old age is the major susceptibility factor. On the contrary, having a cure for aging and refusing to make it available to patients would result in pain and injury, clearly in contradiction with the principle of nonmaleficence ["do no harm"]. Even if we cure aging, individuals will still be able to choose whether they wanted to age or not, in accordance with the principle of respect for autonomy. If someone wants to continue aging despite a cure for aging being available, no one can force him or her not to age. Likewise, if a cure for aging is proven safe and efficient then it should be available to all of those who wish to benefit from it.

Some bioethicists, such as Leon Kass and Francis Fukuyama, argue life-extension is immoral. Of course, since longevity increased 50% in the past century, we may already be living immoral lives just for opposing bacteria, viruses, and cancer when we should let them eat us alive. As I hope I made it clear above, curing aging is ethically the right thing to do.

7

Extending the Human Lifespan Is a Moral Imperative

George Dvorsky

George Dvorsky is the president of the Toronto Transhumanist Association, a nonprofit organization devoted to encouraging the use of technology to transcend the limitations of the human body.

Individuals who oppose scientific advances meant to stop people from aging and dying are not unlike the Luddites, a group of 19th-century British textile workers who broke mechanical looms to protest the advance of industrialization. Today's "bio-Luddites" have an irrational and wrongheaded fear of biotechnology, and if their views gain influence, humans will all be a lot worse off. Efforts to keep science from enhancing and extending the human lifespan amount to little more than a war on life itself. If supported by public policies, these anti-science, pro-death views could lead to such atrocities as the withdrawal of medical care or even government-enforced euthanasia when people reach a maximum allowed age. It is a moral imperative to fight for one's right to live as long as possible.

The late Freddie Mercury of [music group] Queen once asked, "Who wants to live forever?" Pose the question to the growing community of transhumanists, immortalists, cryonicists and various life extension aficionados around the world, and most would surely raise a hand and proclaim, "Uh, that would be me, thank you very much."

George Dvorsky, "Bio-Luddite Nation," The Longevity Meme.org, August 1, 2004. http://www.longevitymeme.org. Reproduced by permission.

Predictably, ever since the mainstream have caught on to such seemingly outlandish desires, life extension advocates have been met with much scorn, ridicule and many rolled eyes—but not for the reasons you might think.

Bio-Luddites—named for their opposition to new biotechnology, such as advanced medical research—certainly don't think that life extension advocates are crazy, at least not about the prospect of life span augmentation and thwarting aging altogether. No, the bio-Luddites are very concerned that this wish might actually come true. The transformation of humans into a deathless species, they argue, could be disastrous on many levels.

As the prospect of radical extension of the healthy human life span becomes more real with each passing year, prominent bio-Luddites have gone on the offensive to convince immortal wannabes that death is where it's at. They speak in a flowery and comforting tone, proclaiming that death defines our species and endows our lives with meaning, purpose and social stability.

The most outspoken of these pro-death advocates are, of course, Leon Kass and Francis Fukuyama, both of whom sit on the President's Council on Bioethics in the US. They're not alone, however, and can count a number of bioconservatives, bioethicists, and other opponents of scientific progress—including Charles Krauthammer and Bill McKibbin—on their side.

I consider myself open to ideas and alternative perspectives, but as I consider the arguments of the bio-Luddites and look deeper into their meaning, I have come to realize that the death-promoting propaganda campaign is more than just a battle for hearts and minds. I get the impression that—should radical life extension technologies become readily available—these detractors, some of whom have the ear of the

President, would go much further than fighting a war of words in their attempt to ensure that we never gain mastery over our mortality.

While the bio-Luddites are directly concerned with the people of the US, encroaching cross-border influences, including the pressure they've put on the United Nations to impose international restrictions on medical research and regenerative medicine, should cause concern for people the world over. So I'm forced to consider what it would take to stop the coming anti-aging revolution, and in doing so I have come to fear the kind of future the bio-Luddites have in mind.

Big Brother Wants You Dead

At times the bio-Luddites sound parochial and authoritarian, and at their worst they sound downright ideological and even totalitarian. Leon Kass has repeatedly stated, "the finitude of human life is a blessing for every individual, whether he knows it or not." And frighteningly, when asked by Brian Alexander, the author of *Rapture: How Biotechnology Became the New Religion*, if the government has a right to tell its citizens that they have to die, Fukuyama answered, frighteningly, "Yes, absolutely."

The demand for a longer, healthier life span is powerful and widespread.

Just what, exactly, does this dynamic duo have in mind for the citizens of the US, and by extension, the rest of the world? I am completely bewildered as to how, at the dawn of the biotech century, such a policy of death by government fiat [decree] could actually be put into place in an ethical, safe and legal manner.

In fact, I believe that it can't. It would take an authoritarian iron fist to stop serious anti-aging efforts—a Brave New

World far scarier than the one that bio-Luddites think the transhumanists and life extension advocates would introduce.

Shame On You for Living

How might this conflict play out? Before the bio-Luddites do anything drastic, they will likely ramp up the pro-death rhetoric to convince people they should abstain from supporting, developing and utilizing life extension technologies. I can already imagine the guilt-tripping psychological warfare. "Die or your children won't be able to find a job," one ad might go.

Realistically, this will have very little impact on public opinions. As demonstrated by the Viagra phenomenon, hormone therapy and a host of other commercially successful products, the demand for a longer, healthier life span is powerful and widespread—even to the point of purchasing unscientific "anti-aging" pills and potions that have no proven effect. Frankly, it is hard to believe that anyone of sound mind and healthy body would see their own death at that very moment in time as "a blessing," no matter how many bioethicists were at hand to convince them of the merits of dying.

The healthy human life span will become increasingly longer, with every year of life bringing people closer to the next medical breakthrough.

Herald Tribune columnist Rich Brooks recently pointed out, "It is death, Kass might say, that gives urgency to life. It drives us to discovery, to cross oceans and reach into the emptiness of space; it is the reason we squeeze pleasure and meaning from every moment and see beauty in every sunset." But if death is such a blessing, asks Brooks, "then why don't we embrace it? Why is life such a desperate enterprise?" Ultimately, says Brooks, "it's because each of us has only one life—a prospect that leads us to live out our lives with meaning and purpose."

And yes, the slope is always slippery. "When disease or hardship strikes, we decide as individuals whether to seek health and life-extending treatment," says Brooks. "Taken collectively, these decisions set the course for humanity. Our collective will to live drives the quest for cures and life-saving technology. Thus taking advantage of medical breakthroughs affirms our humanity rather than diminishing it."

Given the inevitable failure of a pro-death propaganda campaign, the bio-Luddites will have to take their fight to the next level.

Declaring a War on Life

Thanks to the efforts of pioneering biogerontologists such as Aubrey de Grey, Leonard Hayflick and Cynthia Kenyon, aging is increasingly coming to be regarded as a medical condition—a condition that will one day be treated and ultimately cured. Coming from a computer science background, de Grey in particular has demonstrated that aging can be viewed as a solvable engineering problem.

It will only be a matter of time before these and other researchers make greater and greater strides in their work, resulting in a steady flow of life-extending medical interventions destined for the market. The healthy human life span will become increasingly longer, with every year of extra life bringing people closer to the next medical breakthrough. Soon we will achieve "escape velocity," as medical science extends healthy life span faster than we age.

How would we decide what constitutes a life extension intervention? How could we possibly delineate between a therapeutic medical practice and a life extension practice?

This is the vision for the years ahead—unless, of course, drastic measures are put in place to prevent it. Similar to the current War on Drugs, it is conceivable that a government led by bio-Luddites could impose a War on Life, criminalizing and suppressing life extension research. Medical science would be closely monitored and regulated, with researchers forced to work within state-sanctioned guidelines.

This is not as farfetched as it might sound. Current governments in both the US and Canada, for example, have enacted extremely stringent policies in regards to stem cell and cloning research. The US in particular currently boasts one of the most anti-science regimes in all of its history. Given the prominence of religious and Luddite groups, combined with a mostly scientifically illiterate and politically challenged populace, the US government may continue this regressive policy as human enhancement technologies increasingly come into focus and into practical use.

Any policy of enforced euthanasia would be a gross violation of human rights.

Impossible to Enforce

Like the useless, expensive War on Drugs, this War on Life would also have its share of problems and victims. Quelling scientific research into life extension would be exceedingly difficult, creating an enormous black market for researchers, clinicians and therapies—forcing an exodus of scientists to countries with less stringent regulations.

Conservative nations could petition the UN to impose global bans on such research—exactly as they are trying to do now for human therapeutic cloning, with a fair degree of success—but again, imposing and enforcing such a policy would be costly and tragic beyond measure.

Finally, the limits of a war against anti-aging would be impossible to define and circumscribe. Most diseases are caused by aging and the steady deterioration of the body. How would we decide what constitutes a life extension intervention? How could we possibly delineate between a therapeutic medical practice and a life extension practice? Is curing heart disease to be allowed? Diabetes?

Logan's Run

One way around this dilemma for the bio-Luddites would be to enforce a maximum life span. In such a scenario, the elderly would be denied health- and life-extending treatments after passing a certain age. Since it would be impossible to distinguish between any kind of health intervention and life extension, the elderly would simply be left to die.

Society has coped very well . . . by steadily adapting to the realities of longer-lived, healthier citizens.

This reminds me of the campy 1976 sci-fi film *Logan's Run*. The movie takes place in a post-apocalyptic hedonistic world where no one is allowed to live beyond the age of 30. The Orwellian culture is laden with pro-death rhetoric and citizens are made to feel shamed for even thinking about living beyond 30. When their time is up, they're forced to attend a death ritual called "renewal" for the illusory chance of a continued life called "rebirth." If anyone dares to avoid this state-imposed euthanasia, a crime referred to as "running," the offenders are tracked down and mercilessly killed on the spot by "sandmen," a specialty corps put into place for just such purposes.

Quite suddenly, given the stated position of the bio-Luddites, the horror of *Logan's Run* seems a disturbingly real possibility. If, as Fukuyma asserts, the state has the right to tell its citizens that they have to die, and assuming that such a policy would be put in place when life extension technologies arrive—and arrive they will, regardless of propaganda campaigns and draconian anti-science measures—this would seem the only possible recourse to guarantee population turnover.

This begs the question: What would the bio-Luddites set as a maximum allowable life span? How old do people have to be before Leon Kass or Bill McKibbin believes they start to "negatively impact society," families, the "sense of the human life cycle," and "the perception of a fulfilling and meaningful life?" Any decision about a maximum life span would be utterly arbitrary. No figure could ever possibly make sense to everyone or be agreed upon.

Furthermore, any policy of enforced euthanasia would be a gross violation of human rights—the worst and most ethically repugnant thing that most of us could imagine. The elderly would have all the justification in the world to fight against the implementation of state-mandated mass murder. They will continue to have every right for equal access to the best and most effective health interventions that medical science has to offer. In fact, the elderly are already starting to organize and agitate, as recently demonstrated by a group of elderly New Yorkers who openly smuggled drugs from Canada to protest what they see as overly strict and unjust trade regulations.

Worse Than Useless Ethics

Before recorded history began, humans could expect to live just a few years past 30. As recently as a century ago, life expectancy was not much more than 40. Today, the average life span is well into the 70s and creeping into the 80s. People are not just living longer, they're living healthy and vibrantly into their elder years. Today's 70- and 80-year-olds are completely unlike the elderly I remember seeing when I was child growing up in the 1970s.

No one seems to be complaining. In fact, they're celebrating—and rightfully so. Society has coped very well with these changes by steadily adapting to the realities of longer-lived, healthier citizens. The sky hasn't fallen on our heads due to the last 30 extra years of healthy life granted to us—and it won't fall on our heads due to the next 30 either. There's no reason to believe that culture, society and its institutions won't continue to change and adapt to future issues, including any potential overpopulation problems. If past trends are any indication, longer lives in fact mean fewer births and declining population growth.

Meanwhile, pro-death, bio-Luddite bioethicists like Leon Kass and his ilk are offering the worst and most useless kind of ethics. It is an ethics without foundation in reality, devoid of pragmatic guidance and practical solutions. It is an ethics that espouses the enforcement of death on a massive scale. This will not do for the coming realities of 21st century life.

The pro-death rhetoric is only resulting in a confused and scared populace, backwards, stifling legislation and a depraved indifference to the ongoing toll of 50 million lives lost each year. Since the members of the US President's Council on Bioethics have declared their recognition of the scientific plausibility of serious anti-aging research, their systematic curtailment and prevention of this research could be construed someday as a crime against humanity.

Don't believe their hype. Fight for your right to live.

8

Life-Extension Technologies Can Be Misused

Leon R. Kass

Leon R. Kass is the former chair of the President's Council on Bioethics and is a Hertog fellow at the American Enterprise Institute, a conservative think tank.

The advances in biomedical science that are developed as well-intentioned treatments for diseases and to increase longevity have a dark side as well. Such therapeutic technologies can be misused to enhance, extend and perfect human life in ways that are often frivolous, sometimes deeply troubling, and occasionally frightening. It is already clear that recent gains in health and longevity have created the demand for more and more ways to unnaturally enhance the human condition. It is inevitable that as new technologies emerge, they will be misused as well. The ideal human life is not one lived with an ageless body or with help from science to supplement physical abilities and transcend human limitations. Rather, it is a life lived in close contact with the rhythms of nature and with the awareness of time itself as a necessary player in human destiny. It is important to resist the seductive promises of technological perfection.

As nearly everyone appreciates, we live near the beginning of the golden age of biotechnology. For the most part, we should be mightily glad that we do. We and our friends and loved ones are many times over the beneficiaries of its cures

Leon R. Kass, "Beyond Therapy: Biotechnology and the Pursuit of Human Improvement," Presented to the President's Council on Bioethics to Aid Discussion, January 2003. http://www.bioethics.gov.

for diseases, prolongation of life, and amelioration of suffering, psychic as well as somatic. We should be deeply grateful for the gifts of human ingenuity and cleverness and for the devoted efforts of scientists, physicians, and entrepreneurs who have used these gifts to make those benefits possible. And, mindful that modern biology is just entering puberty, we suspect that we ain't seen nothin' yet.

Yet, notwithstanding these blessings, present and projected, we have also seen more than enough to make us anxious and concerned. For we recognize that the powers made possible by biomedical science can be used for non-therapeutic purposes, serving ends that range from the frivolous and disquieting to the offensive and pernicious. These powers are available as instruments of bioterrorism (e.g., genetically engineered drug-resistant bacteria, or drugs that obliterate memory); as agents of social control (e.g., drugs to tame rowdies, or fertility blockers for welfare recipients); and as means of trying to improve or perfect our bodies and minds and those of our children (e.g., genetically engineered supermuscles, or drugs to improve memory). Anticipating possible threats to our security, freedom, and even our very humanity, many people are increasingly worried about where biotechnology may be taking us. We are concerned about what others might do to us, but also about what we might do to ourselves. We are concerned that our society might be harmed and that we ourselves might be diminished, indeed, in ways that could undermine the highest and richest possibilities of human life. . . .

I want to discuss only the last and most seductive of these disquieting prospects—the use of biotechnical powers to pursue "perfection," both of body and of mind. I do so partly because it is the most neglected topic in public and professional bioethics, yet it is I believe the deepest source of public anxiety, represented in the concern about "man playing God," or about the Brave New World or a "post-human future." It raises the weightiest questions of bioethics, touching on the ends and goals of the biomedical enterprise, the nature and meaning of human flourishing, and the intrinsic threat of dehumanization (or the promise of super-humanization). It compels attention to what it means to be a human being and to be active as a human being. And it gets us beyond our narrow preoccupation with the "life issues" of abortion or embryo destruction, important though they are, to deal with what is genuinely novel and worrisome in the biotechnical revolution: not the old crude power to kill the creature made in God's image, but the science-based sophisticated power to remake him after our own fantasies.

Even the bizarre prospect of machine-brain interaction and implanted nanotechnological devices starts with therapeutic efforts to enable the blind to see and the deaf to hear.

Biotechnology Raises Complicated Issues

This is, to be sure, a very difficult topic and one not obviously relevant to current public policy debate. Compared with other contemporary issues in bioethics, the questions connected with biotechnological enhancement seem abstract, remote, and too philosophical, unfit for political or other action. The concerns it raises are also complicated and inchoate, hard to formulate in general terms, especially because the differing technologically based powers raise different ethical and social questions. Finally, bothering oneself about this semi-futuristic prospect of interest to prosperous Americans seems even to me precious and a touch self-indulgent, given that we live in a world in which millions are dying annually of malaria, AIDS, and malnutrition for want (in part) of more essential biotechnologies, and many of our fellow Americans lack basic health care. Yet this push toward bio-engineered perfection strikes me as the wave of the future, one that will sneak up on us before we know it and, if we are not careful, sweep us up and tow us under. For we can already see how the recent gains in health and longevity have produced not contentment but rather an increased appetite for more. And, from recent trends in the medicalization of psychiatry and the study of the mind, it seems clear that the expected new discoveries about the workings of the psyche and the biological basis of behavior will greatly increase the ability to alter and the temptation to improve them. Besides, policy decisions we today are making—for instance, what to do about human cloning or sex selection and genetic selection of embryos, or whether to get comfortable prescribing psychotropic drugs to 3-year-olds, or how vigorously to pursue research into the biology of senescence—will shape the world of the future for people who will not have chosen to live under its utopia-seeking possibilities. It is up to us now to begin thinking about these matters.

Defining the Concerns

What exactly are the powers that I am talking about? What kind of technologies makes them possible? What sorts of ends are they likely to serve? How soon are they available? They are powers that affect the capacities and activities of the human body, powers that affect the capacities and activities of the mind or soul, and powers that affect the shape of the human lifecycle, at both ends and in between. We already have powers to prevent fertility and to promote it; to initiate life in the laboratory; to screen our genes, both as adults and as embryos, and to select (or reject) nascent life based on genetic criteria; to insert new genes into various parts of the adult body, and someday soon also into gametes and embryos; to enhance muscle performance and endurance; to replace body parts with natural or mechanical organs, and perhaps soon, to wire ourselves using computer chips implanted into the body and brain; to alter memory, mood, and attention though psychoactive drugs; and to prolong not just the average but also the maximum human life expectancy. The technologies for altering our native capacities are mainly those of genetic screening and genetic engineering; drugs, especially psychoactive ones; and the ability to replace body parts or to insert novel ones. The availability of some of these capacities, using these techniques, has been demonstrated only with animals; but others are already in use in humans.

It bears emphasis that these powers have not been developed for the purpose of producing perfect or post-human beings. They have been produced largely for the purpose of preventing and curing disease, and of reversing disabilities. Even the bizarre prospect of machine-brain interaction and implanted nanotechnological devices starts with therapeutic efforts to enable the blind to see and the deaf to hear. Yet the "dual use" aspects of most of these powers, encouraged by the ineradicable human urge toward "improvement" and the commercial interests that see market opportunities for non-therapeutic uses, means that we must not be lulled to sleep by the fact that the originators of these powers were no friends to Brave New World. Once here, techniques and powers can produce desires where none existed before, and things often go where no one ever intended. . . .

The pursuit of an ageless body is . . . a distraction and a deformation.

Some Examples

To make a bit more concrete the prospects for pursuing these goals, I offer you some technological innovations that, in varying degrees, can serve the purposes. With respect to the pursuit of "ageless bodies," we can replace worn out parts, we can improve upon normal and healthy parts, and, more radically, we can try to retard or stop the entire process of biological senescence [aging]. With respect to the first, please keep in mind organ transplantation and the prospect of re-generative medicine where decayed tissues are replaced with new ones produced from stem cells. With respect to the second, consider precise genetic modification of muscles, through a single injection of a growth factor gene, that keep the trans-formed muscles whole, vigorous, and free of age-related de-cline (powers already used to produce mighty mouse and su-per rat, and soon to be available for treatment of muscular dystrophy and muscle weakness in the elderly but also of in-terest to football coaches and to the hordes of people who spend two hours daily pumping iron and sculpting their "abs"). And with respect to the last, keep in mind recent dis-coveries in the genetics of aging that have shown how the maximum lifespan of worms and flies can be increased two- and three-fold by alterations in a single gene, a gene now known to be present also in mammals.

With respect to the pursuit of "happy souls," we can elimi-nate psychic distress, we can produce states of transient eu-phoria, and we can engineer more permanent conditions of good cheer, optimism, and contentment. Accordingly, please keep in mind drugs now available that, administered promptly at the time of memory formation, blunt markedly the painful emotional content of the newly formed memories of trau-matic events (so-called "memory erasure," a remedy being sought to prevent post-traumatic stress disorder). Keep in mind, second, simple euphoriants, like Ecstasy, the forerunner of Huxley's "soma," widely used on college campuses; and, fi-nally, powerful yet seemingly safe anti-depressant and mood brighteners like Prozac, capable in some people of utterly changing their outlook on life from that of Eeyore to that of Mary Poppins. . . .

Living Involves the Entire Lifecycle

Let me suggest . . . that a flourishing human life is not a life lived with an ageless body or untroubled soul, but rather a life lived in rhythmned time, mindful of time's limits, appreciative of each season and filled first of all with those intimate human relations that are ours only because we are born, age, replace ourselves, decline, and die—and know it. It is a life of aspiration, made possible by and borne of experienced lack, of the disproportion between the transcendent longings of the soul and the limited capacities of our bodies and minds. It is a life that stretches toward some fulfillment to which our natural human soul has been oriented, and, unless we extirpate the source, will always be oriented. It is a life not of better genes and enhancing chemicals but of love and friendship, song and dance, speech and deed, working and learning, revering and worshipping. The pursuit of an ageless body is finally a distraction and a deformation. The pursuit of an untroubled and self-satisfied soul is deadly to desire. Finitude recognized spurs aspiration. Fine aspiration acted upon *is itself* the core of happiness. Not the agelessness of the body nor the contentment of the soul nor even the list of external achievement and accomplishments of life, but the engaged and energetic being-at-work of what nature uniquely gave to us is what we need to treasure and defend against the devilish promise of technological perfection.

9

Science Should Extend the Human Lifespan Indefinitely

Aubrey de Grey

Aubrey de Grey is the chairman and chief science officer of the Methuselah Foundation, a nonprofit organization committed to finding a cure for age-related disease, disability, suffering, and death.

For most of human history, lifespans were relatively short and most people died from causes unrelated to aging. In today's industrialized world, however, people live much longer—so much so that aging eventually kills around 90 percent of the population. This is because the biological changes associated with aging underlie most diseases. It makes no sense, then, that medical science and public policy focus all of their research efforts and funding on diseases such as cancer and heart disease, rather than seeking a cure for aging. Aging should be seen as a disease in itself. Preventing the suffering and death that are the direct consequences of the aging process is well worth any societal consequences that might arise. The only ethical thing that science can do is pursue a cure for aging so that life can be extended as long as possible.

It has been obvious to me since my earliest days that the eventually fatal physiological decline associated with getting older is both tragic and potentially preventable by medical intervention. It was, therefore, a matter of some consternation

Aubrey de Grey, "Old People Are People Too: Why It Is Our Duty to Fight Aging to the Death," *Cato Unbound*, December 2007. Republished with permission of Cato Institute, conveyed through Copyright Clearance Center, Inc.

to me to discover in my late twenties that my view on this matter was not universally shared. In this essay I explode various myths and illogicalities that surround the effort to combat (and especially to defeat) aging, with an emphasis on some that are often perpetrated by currently influential commentators.

A pro-aging message . . . is a crutch, allowing its recipients to divert their attention to less unsavory matters.

Cancer is undesirable. Heart disease is undesirable. So are type 2 diabetes, Alzheimer's and a thousand other debilitations that predominantly afflict those over the age of 40. Is it not then bizarre that we should have any hesitation in declaring that aging in general, being the molecular and cellular root cause of all these phenomena, is just as deserving of the attention of our medical research efforts?

There is, in fact, a simple psychological explanation. Until very recently, aging has been regarded by all credentialed biogerontologists as far too complex to be substantially postponed within the lifetime of anyone currently alive. Indeed, this remains the majority view, with the present author one of a still rather small (though growing) minority who perceive a way forward. This being so, it makes good psychological sense to find some way to convince oneself that aging is all for the best, and thus to put it out of one's mind, rather than to spend one's life preoccupied with one's grisly and inescapable fate. The fact that such rationalizations are stunningly irrational from a purely objective standpoint is irrelevant.

The Pro-aging Myth

Unfortunately, irrational rationalizations only work for as long as we can suspend our disbelief. As a result, some of the world's finest minds have gained great prominence by articulating excuses for aging that sound convincing to those desperate to be convinced. A pro-aging message presented as a moral or sociological *fait accompli* [irreversible fact] is a crutch, allowing its recipients to divert their attention to less unsavory matters.

Apologists for aging are often keen to cast the wish for a longer life as an ignoble, even unmanly desire.

But, of course, the authors of these arguments don't see it that way—not least because they believe their own arguments just as sincerely as their followers do. Hence the rest of this essay.

In the Greek myth of Tithonus, the (mortal) eponymous Trojan warrior won the heart of the (immortal) goddess Eos. Being too junior a deity to be able to immortalize her lover, Eos asked Zeus to do this—but "forgot" to ask that Tithonus also be eternally youthful. He thus became ever more frail and decrepit, such that eventually Eos had no choice but to turn him into a grasshopper.

The survival of this myth is a shining example of the pro-aging trance in action. The idea that a postponement of death might occur without a postponement of aging is plainly arbitrary (as well as biomedically absurd—being frail is risky and always will be), yet it is the presumption made unquestioningly in the story—and, as those who have raised such matters with the public know well, equally unquestioningly in the knee-jerk reactions of many when called upon to contemplate radical life extension.

Why Postpone Aging?

Erudite commentators tend to avoid this error in its grossest form, but subtler versions of it abound. The most dangerous one is with regard to the *motivation* for intervening in aging. Let us consider some reasons why one might want to postpone aging:

1. to live longer
2. to let others live longer
3. to avoid debilitation/disease/dependency in later life
4. to let others avoid debilitation/disease/dependency in later life

---

The only realistic approach to greatly postponing bad deaths is to combat aging itself.

Even once it is accepted that the postponement of death will probably be achieved only by the corresponding postponement of frailty, apologists for aging are often keen to cast the wish for a longer life as an ignoble, even unmanly desire. The controversial nature of this starting point has an insidiously indirect effect: it distracts attention from the fact that even if this wish *were* ignoble, the conclusion that we should not strive to defeat aging does not follow. The unstated assumption in this form of the Tithonus error is twofold: firstly that those who wish for aging to be defeated wish it for the putatively ignoble first reason, rather than for the more unassailably noble others, and secondly that the merits of such-and-such a future scenario depend on why people strove to bring it about. I myself am much less motivated to combat aging by selfish desire than by humanitarian incentives, not least because I know that I can only alter the life expectancy of a particular individual (myself, say) by a small amount through my actions, whereas on a global scale I may save a phenomenal number of lives. But even if most pro-longevists *were* driven by a personal desire to live for centuries, and even if for the sake of argument we were to agree that this is not a noble motive, so what? Good deeds done for "invalid" reasons are still good deeds.

Biomedical Wishful Thinking

There once was a time when most deaths were from causes unrelated to aging—predation, starvation, hypothermia, etc.

In today's industrialized world, such deaths are in the minority: aging kills around 90% of us. But some deaths from aging are widely held to be worse than others. Particular importance is often attached to the amount of time spent in a frail state before death: dying in one's sleep in the absence of chronic disease and at an age somewhat (but not too much!) in excess of the prevailing average is considered "a good death" with which doctors should perhaps not interfere, whereas the protracted suffering endured by many elderly today (especially with the rise of Alzheimer's disease) is a worthy target of medical intervention. This leads to the refrain that we should prioritize "giving life to years, not just years to life." As with the Tithonus error above, this position is predicated on a miasma [a poisonous atmosphere] of arbitrary assumptions and distractions.

Firstly, it is distinctly unclear whether a sick person's life is any less valuable (hence, worthy of sustaining) than a robust person's. After all, no less an icon of contemporary moral philosophy than President George W. Bush stated in connection with the [Terri] Schiavo case [which involved the legality of removing a feeding tube from someone in a persistent vegetative state] that "it is wise to always err on the side of life." Note again the paradoxical utility of a controversial aspect of a position in distracting attention from aspects that are more unequivocally indefensible.

The question humanity must face up to is clear: is the prevention of the suffering currently associated with most deaths from old age valuable enough to justify the inevitable side effect of radically increased lifespans?

Secondly, the views of the victim of a "good death" tend to be forgotten once that death has occurred. Prevailing quality of life (and perception of near-term future quality) bears heavily on many people's interest in self-preservation—and why should it not?—so those who have been getting quite a lot out of life right up until last night might, were their opinion sought, hesitate to join the consensus that it wasn't such a bad thing that they didn't wake up this morning.

Thirdly, the Tithonus error is equally erroneous when inverted. Just as being frail is risky, so being robust is not risky: people who are not in the advanced stages of one or another age-related disease will mostly not die until they are, whatever their chronological age. . . . There are, of course, easy ways to change that—discontinue the supply of influenza jabs to the elderly, for example—but such approaches have not found favor with the general public (nor, it might be noted, with geronto-apologists) in the past and show no sign of doing so in the future.

Delaying Death Means Increasing Life Expectancy

The practical fact is that, of the three categories of death enumerated at the beginning of this section (early, "bad" late and "good" late), society seems committed to delaying all three. The only issue is the relative priority that should be given to delaying one versus another—and this must be evaluated in the context of foreseeable biomedical reality, not fantasy. Specifically, those who fear the consequences of a dramatic delay in both types of late death are engaging in profound intellectual dishonesty if they ignore the fact that meaningful compression of morbidity—that is, selective postponement of bad death and consequent increase in good deaths, without much change in life expectancy—is biomedically implausible. Rather, they must accept the fact that the only realistic approach to greatly postponing bad deaths is to combat aging itself, and that this will correspondingly postpone good deaths, thereby—unless we deliberately eschew measures to prevent early deaths, as noted above—greatly raising life expectancy, with all that that entails.

The question that humanity must face up to is clear: is the prevention of the suffering currently associated with most deaths from old age valuable enough to justify the inevitable side effect of radically increased lifespans? The question is not whether that side effect is good or bad—a question on which opinions will surely remain divided for some time to come. The question, rather, is whether that side effect is *so* bad as to outweigh the benefits of eliminating aging-related suffering. Dodging this question is unacceptable—and thus, for those who profess to dispense wisdom on ethical matters, it is unforgivable.

The Feasibility and Desirability Argument

Suppose we were to devise a feasible anti-aging intervention that, once developed, would postpone both good and bad late deaths by a modest but non-trivial amount—ten or twenty years, say. Suppose, further, that both the development and the provision of this intervention were very expensive. The ethical arguments against such expenditure are far more reasonable than those that I have demolished above. Specifically, one might point to the much more limited improvement in overall quality of life (because, since early deaths would still be in the minority, the average time spent debilitated before death would be unchanged). One might defensibly conclude that the societal drawbacks of such a measure—increasing the rich/poor health divide, in particular—outweighed these much more modest health benefits, and even the very large economic benefits of keeping the population healthy for longer.

This has proven an irresistible temptation to gerontoapologists, and the following script has been repeated ad nauseam. When presented with the moral unassailability of the quest to defeat aging entirely, they overwhelmingly present arguments against *modest* postponement of aging instead, quietly eliding [leaving out] the distinction and portraying the reality as the worst of both worlds (the downsides of radical life extension with only the upsides of modest life extension). When confronted with their error, they retort that dramatic postponement (even defeat) of aging is "clearly" infeasible and thus not an appropriate topic for discussion. When it is pointed out that their certitude on this matter belies the fact that they are bioethicists, not biogerontologists, they point to the clear consensus of public statements of biogerontologists, which indeed centers on the feasibility of modest life extension but the infeasibility of defeating aging. When reminded that biogerontologists would say that, wouldn't they (since they are funded mainly by taxpayers, who suffer from the pro-aging trance that conservative bioethicists work so hard to perpetuate) reply that the existence of bad reasons to say something doesn't imply the non-existence of valid reasons. When directed to the concerted and spectacularly unsuccessful attempts made by vested-interest-driven prominent biogerontologists to explain to neutral experts why the defeat of aging is infeasible they merely repeat the same reply—for that is all they have.

This tactic can be summed up succinctly. Geronto-apologists simultaneously hold, and alternately express, the following two positions:

- They refuse to consider seriously whether defeating aging is feasible, because they are sure it would not be desirable;

- They refuse to consider seriously whether defeating aging is desirable, because they are sure it is not feasible.

Like a child hiding in a double-doored wardrobe, they cower behind one door when the other is opened, then dash to the other when it is closed and before the first is opened. Only when both doors are flung open in unison is their hiding place revealed. They are both well and truly open now, and the time when this sleight of hand was effective has passed.

Fearmongering and Implausible Deniability

A venerable rhetorical tactic in the promotion of fragile positions is to raise in the audience's mind the specter of some terrible consequence of the opposing position without actually spelling it out. Unnerving questions are asked—but then, rather than answers offered, the subject is changed, leaving the concern to fester in the subconscious. The author escapes, however, with the knowledge that if challenges are raised to the validity of these concerns he can resort to the claim that he never actually said that.

The fact that efforts to postpone human aging will definitely not bear much fruit for at least a few decades is held as a reason to deprioritize such efforts in favor of combating already preventable problems.

This tactic has been all too evident in prominent analyses of whether we should combat aging. I will use as my illustration the chapter "Ageless Bodies" from the President's Council report *Beyond Therapy*, but readers will notice abundant echoes of other writings. The litany of obfuscation begins by exploiting the terminological ambiguity of the word "ageless" with observations such as "An ageless body is almost a contradiction in terms, since all physical things necessarily decay over time." Many pages are then devoted to detailed discussion of various age-retarding measures that have already been demonstrated in the laboratory, without mention of the fact that no credentialed biogerontologist currently claims that any such technique will ever deliver genuine agelessness.

By contrast, no space whatever is given to the work being done on bona fide regenerative medicine, which is the only approach that truly does have such potential. This confusion is amplified when ethical matters are turned to, e.g. with the stage set by declaring that the idea is to extend the working lifetime of all bodily functions by the same *finite* amount (thus allowing the fear to be raised that some would be extended longer than others). Then the fearmongering can begin in earnest. Preposterous propositions such as that "Our dedication to our activities, our engagement with life's callings and our continued interest in our projects all rely to some degree upon a sense that we are giving of ourselves, in a process destined to result in our complete expenditure" are articulated; but then, rather than being quixotically defended (and their absurdity thus exposed), they are sidestepped—"This is not to say that [a life lived devoid of that sense] will be worse—but it will very likely be quite different"—and a new topic hastily begun. The same tactic is repeated over and over again: boredom, childlessness, meaning, families, creativity and more are introduced and then left hanging, with no explicit conclusions asserted, thus distracting the reader from the text's naked bias of emphasis of the risks of radical life extension over the benefits. . . .

Urgency, Reflective Equilibrium, and Repugnance

When thoroughly cornered on the question of whether the defeat of aging would be a good thing, geronto-apologists generally turn as a last resort to the cry "Okay, but first things first!" The fact that efforts to postpone human aging will definitely not bear much fruit for at least a few decades is held as a reason to deprioritize such efforts in favor of combating already preventable problems.

It is trivial to expose the ethical bankruptcy of this position. We lock people up for the same amount of time if they kill people with a gun or with a booby-trap bomb, even though the interval between the murderer's action and the victim's death differs by several orders of magnitude in the two cases. The same irrelevance of that interval applies to the saving of lives, since action and inaction are morally indistinguishable. We are close enough today to defeating aging that serendipity does not define the timeframe: the sooner and harder we try to do it, the sooner we'll succeed. Thus, our inaction today costs lives—lots of lives.

Old people are people too, so aging must be seen for what it is: a scourge that deprives far more people of far more healthy years than any other.

Time was when we didn't lock people up for either such crime: we executed them. That tradition has been roundly rejected across almost the entire developed world, as have slavery, sexism, racism, faithism, homophobia—and, with the notable exception of this essay's subject, ageism. Our view of what is and is not repugnant evolves by a process best described by [American philosopher John] Rawls, with the name "reflective equilibrium," in which logical contradictions between simultaneously held values are progressively highlighted and resolved by the abandonment of the less central one.

Old People Are People Too

[Bioethicist Leon] Kass has courageously defended an academically unfashionable position that I personally share, which ethicists call "non-cognitivism" and he called "the wisdom of repugnance." In this view, one's gut feeling regarding the ethical status of an action is not something to be meekly subordinated to logic, because the very existence of that feeling constitutes evidence of its ethical correctness. However, the beauty of reflective equilibrium is that it works for cognitivists and non-cognitivists alike: one needs no belief in the existence of objective morality to appreciate that one's moral stance on all matters should be logically consistent.

Thus, it is the duty of opinion-formers on ethical matters to work to accelerate the reflective equilibrium process: to identify and highlight internal contradictions in conventional moral wisdom so that the competing views can battle it out.

In the case of radical life extension, since the equivalences noted above (action/inaction, ageism/discrimination, saving/ extending lives) are so fundamental, the odds are rather heavily stacked against the pro-aging position's survival of this process. The title of this essay really says it all: discrimination of any sort is passé. Old people are people too, so aging must be seen for what it is: a scourge that deprives far more people of far more healthy years than any other. Aging, in a word, is re-pugnant, and we would be wiser to follow Kass's general maxim than his specific conclusion. To persist in defending aging is psychologically excusable—fear of the unknown is a reasonable emotion, in particular—but it is ethically inexcus-able.

10

Science Would Be Wrong to Extend Life Indefinitely

Diana Schaub

Diana Schaub is a professor of political science at Loyola College in Maryland and a member of the Hoover Institution Task Force on the Virtues of a Free Society.

While living forever, or at least a lot longer, might sound attractive, it actually would be a negative thing both for individuals and for society. A 1,000-year lifespan would introduce a variety of undesirable personal, social, and political consequences. For example, because a human life would be so much longer than that of an animal such as a dog, humans might find themselves avoiding contact with other creatures because of the seemingly never-ending cycle of loss. Human relationships would certainly also be affected. The marriage vows of "till death do us part" would take on a whole new gravity, and couples who might remain together for 30 years for the sake of the kids probably won't do so for 300. Extended life also translates to the possibility of extended tyrannies, as brutal and authoritarian leaders would live for centuries rather than decades. Science would be wrong to take humanity into this territory.

Do not go gentle into that good
night,

Old age should burn and rave at
close of day;

Diana Schaub, "Ageless Mortals," *Cato Unbound*, December 5, 2007. Republished with permission of Cato Institute, conveyed through Copyright Clearance Center, Inc.

Rage, rage against the dying of the
light.

—Dylan Thomas

A ubrey de Grey doesn't promise that the lights won't go
out, but he does think we may be able to change when
and how they go out. He rages not at death but decline. Of
course, if bodily decline can be successfully staved off, then a
major cause of death will have been removed. Accordingly, de
Grey envisions a future where the human lifespan will be
"radically increased." Although his present essay is oddly reti-
cent about attaching a number to the word "radically," the
website of de Grey's Methuselah Foundation is more forth-
right. The Bible puts Methuselah's age at 969 years and de
Grey is confident that science could restore such antediluvian
longevity to humankind. He calls for a life-prolongation
project that would deliver a 1,000-year human lifespan. Pre-
sumably, life would still be cut short either by events that continue to elude rational control—accidents, acts of God (like
the flood that did in Methuselah), and acts of others (war and
murder)—or, I suppose, by deliberate choice, whether heroic
self-sacrifice or suicide. So, we won't be deathless, but we will
be ageless (or pretty nearly so). Death will come, but not as a
predictable culmination of a life cycle.

Radical and Visionary

De Grey's thought has the distinct advantage of being vision-
ary and radical. The boldness of his forecasting invites equally
far-reaching speculations (including some forebodings) about
the character and shape of human lives measured in centuries
rather than decades. Before I say "yes" to a whole lot more
life, I would want to think about the relation between more
life and a good life. I must admit that I don't find persuasive
de Grey's attempt to silence potential doubters and dissenters
by brandishing the specter of age-discrimination and insisting

on "our duty." If the powerful desire for self-preservation, coupled with the fear of death, is not enough to fill the anti-aging ranks, I don't think calls to duty will do it.

After all, most of us—so long as we're not environmentalists of the humanity-hating stripe—already have pretty pronounced pro-longevity sympathies. Over the last century, there have been tremendous gains in average life expectancy throughout the developed world. In the United States, for instance, the figure went from 48 to 78 as a result of reductions in infant mortality and other causes of premature death. Similar improvements in nutrition, safety, and longevity are earnestly being sought in less developed nations. At the same time, scientists and doctors are searching for cures for the diseases that afflict us in later life. All of this is welcome. Right now, the human lifespan is 122 years (maximum lifespan is set by the longest-lived individual of a species). You might say we are endeavoring to make life expectancy approximate lifespan. To the extent that we can close that gap, human beings could expect to live long and relatively healthy lives.

How would one feel at, say, 370 years of age, contemplating pet number 30-something?

I suspect that de Grey is correct that in the course of this desirable work to allow us to live out our natural lifespan, we will increasingly turn our attention to the mysteries of aging. We will seek to arrest or even defeat senescence [aging]. Age-retardation techniques, whatever they may be (candidates at this point include caloric restriction, genetic manipulation, regenerative medicine, antioxidants, and manipulation of hormones and telomeres), will open the prospect of re-engineering the human lifespan. This is an altogether different prospect—not a modest postponement of aging, but a dramatic one.

The 1,000-Year Lifespan

I don't know whether a 1,000-year lifespan is scientifically feasible, but I'm quite willing to grant for the purposes of the argument that it is. More interesting, at least for a political scientist with a humanities bent, is whether it's desirable. The cliché one often heard about Marxist communism was that it "sounds good in theory, but won't work in practice"—in other words, that it was desirable, but not feasible. I always thought the cliché had it backwards. It was the communist dream itself that was undesirable. Sitting here with an aching back and my share of middle-aged complaints, I'm not quite willing to say that agelessness is undesirable but, on the other hand, I can't shake the conviction that the achievement of a 1,000-year lifespan would produce a dystopia. Our moral obligations to posterity require us to give more comprehensive thought to what we bequeath them—not merely physically, but psychologically and politically.

If there are trade-offs between long life and new life, then the quest for individual immortality may pose dangers for the well-being of the human collective, whether at the level of family, the nation, or the species.

De Grey singles out for criticism the "Ageless Bodies" chapter in *Beyond Therapy: Biotechnology and the Pursuit of Happiness*. He faults the President's Council on Bioethics for asking questions—"unnerving questions" that "fester in the audience's mind." To my mind, unnerving questions are the stuff of philosophic inquiry. We should wonder about the effects of a 1,000-year lifespan on the "moral contents of life."

Let me start my own speculations with what might seem a frivolous topic: pet dogs. For those who love their dogs, the disproportion between the human and canine lifespan is already painful. I know of dog-lovers who just can't bring themselves to get a new puppy after they've lost one too many.

How would one feel at, say, 370 years of age, contemplating pet number 30-something? The physical energy required for a new puppy is nothing compared to the psychic energy. So, I don't think it's absurd to worry about the effects of extremely long life on our commitments, aspirations, and receptivity to new life and love.

Personal, Social, and Political Consequences

Perhaps we won't find it disturbing to be so out of sync with the rest of creation (particularly not if we take a chosen few, like our dogs, with us into hyper-longevity). Our human companions, in any case, would be equally long-lived. But how would human relations be affected? How would monogamy fare? It's not doing great as it is, but could one even imagine the vow "till death do us part" when death might be nine centuries away? If monogamy simply disappears as a promise and an expectation, we might be confronted with the human version of the puppy problem: would there be enough psychic energy for ever-renewed love? Life takes its toll on the spirit as well as the body. What would the tally of disappointments, betrayals, and losses be over a millennium? Would we love other people more or less than at present? Would we be better partners, parents, friends, and neighbors? What would it be like to experience the continued vitality of the body in conjunction with the aging of the spirit? Would it mean the best of both worlds: the vitality of youth with the wisdom of maturity? Or the worst of both worlds: the characteristic vices of age with the strength of will to impose them on others?

The consequences of radical life-prolongation would not be purely individual, but social and political as well. Since tyranny is an aspiration coeval [existing with] with political life, we might wonder what the effects of millennial existence would be on the possibilities of tyranny. Every era so far has generated instances of life-long rule—of tyrants who die in their beds having quashed all hope of liberty during their lifetimes. Would a 1,000-year lifespan also mean 1,000 years of the likes of Stalin—a Stalin who perhaps uses agelessness (and other biotech discoveries) as a tool of political control?

Even without the threat of vastly extended tyranny, a nation of ageless individuals could well produce a sclerotic [hardened] society, petrified in its ways and views. Senescence escorts us, more or less gracefully, off the stage, making room for fresh generations. The aging of individuals may be one condition for societal renascence [rebirth]. Fascinatingly, longevity research in animals suggests that one cost of age-retardation is sterility or decreased fertility. If there are trade-offs between long life and new life, then the quest for individual immortality may pose dangers for the well-being of the human collective, whether at the level of the family, the nation, or the species. While frailty and finitude don't seem such good things, they may be inextricably entwined with other very good things that we would not want to sacrifice.

11

Life Extension Widens the Gap Between Rich and Poor

Melissa Fusco

Melissa Fusco was a 2006 science-writing intern at Stanford News Service, an information service of Stanford University.

It seems clear that the human lifespan will soon be dramatically extended by modern medicine. Widespread use of anti-aging technologies will create a variety of social and economic challenges. Between 2010 and 2030, the most common age of death will jump by 20 years—five times faster than the current rate of increase. Such a significant population shift will be difficult for many countries to handle. Most troubling is the longevity gap that may form between rich and poor countries and individuals as the wealthy enjoy access to life-extending health care that the poor cannot afford. The current lack of antiretroviral drugs to combat AIDS in Africa while the West has a steady supply is a stark example of the kind of disparity that could arise over life-extension technologies. It is essential to consider these challenges now and prepare for them rather than be surprised by their impact at a later time.

In the 21st century, state-of-the-art anti-aging technologies may extend human lifespans at an unprecedented rate, bringing with them a host of social and economic challenges, says biologist Shripad Tuljapurkar of Stanford University.

The combined impact of these medical advances would have major implications for the global community in the new

Melissa Fusco, "World Faces Challenge as Technologies Lengthen Life Expectancies, Biologist Says," Stanford Report, March 1, 2006. http://news-service.stanford.edu. Copyright © 2006 Stanford University. Reproduced by permission.

century. Tuljapurkar, the Dean and Virginia Morrison Professor of Population Studies, will give a talk Feb. 17 on the demographic and economic consequences of anti-aging therapies at the annual meeting of the American Association of Science in St. Louis.

"Some people believe we are on the brink of being able to extend human lifespan significantly, because we've got most of the technologies we need to do it," Tuljapurkar said.

There is hope in the scientific community that extending life also will prolong the healthy and active years of life, he said, adding, "That's where I come in."

Aging Populations Around the World

In his research, Tuljapurkar selected representative populations from different countries around the world and examined relationships between historical trends in aging, population growth and economic activity. His analysis combined these data with forecasts on the future of anti-aging treatments from leading researchers in the field.

The result? "We've come up with a scenario: Starting around 2010, we could see lifespan increase dramatically," he predicted.

Even countries with stable populations will see the age composition of the citizenry undergo a dramatic shift toward the elderly, who are frequently retired or disabled.

Tuljapurkar estimated that between 2010 and 2030, the modal, or most common, age of death will increase by 20 years if anti-aging therapies come into widespread use. This projected increase reflects a lifespan growth rate that is five times faster than the current rate, increasing the modal age of death in industrialized countries such as the United States from roughly 80 years to 100.

"We studied different countries around the world that are representative of different situations and took a look at where they'd end up," Tuljapurkar said. "One thing that happens right away, which nobody seems to have thought of, is that the total global population increases dramatically. From an original projection of 8 billion we end up topping out at 10 to 11 billion. In many countries, this would have an enormous, and not necessarily positive, impact. For example, the idea that China would go from 1.5 to 1.8 billion, just because of this, is a bit frightening."

On the other hand, he said, a longer-lived population could be good news for many European countries with low fertility rates. "Countries like Sweden and Italy have been having this huge debate for many years over population decline," Tuljapurkar explained. "A lot of the debate is about immigration: People have been telling them they need to increase immigration in order to keep the economy going."

However, an increase in citizenry is only one factor in determining a nation's socioeconomic health, he noted. Even countries with stable populations will see the age composition of the citizenry undergo a dramatic shift toward the elderly, who are frequently retired or disabled.

The lifespan boom will be confined to wealthy countries, where citizens can afford anti-aging technology.

To factor in this phenomenon, Tuljapurkar examined the effects of anti-aging technologies on the national dependency ratio—the proportion of retired people (age 65 and over) to working people (age 20–65) in a population. This ratio is a crucial factor in determining Medicare and Social Security policies in the United States, he said.

Current worries over the fate of Social Security center on the impending retirement of the Baby Boom generation. By 2035, the U.S. dependency ratio is projected to double from approximately 1:5 to just above 2:5. Increased boomer lifespans will add an alarming extra weight to an already sagging system. Factoring in increased lifespans, Tuljapurkar calculated that current forecasts for dependency ratios could fall short by a factor of two—meaning that in America, the ratio will actually quadruple to 4:5.

"It's staggering to think about the fiscal effects of this," he said.

Inequality

The situation is equally troubling on a global scale. While science may be on the brink of unlocking the mysteries of the aging process, Tuljapurkar is worried that the world is unprepared for the inequalities that this new knowledge may generate between the world's rich and poor.

"Are some people going to be left behind? Are we going to make society far more unequal than it is now?" he asked. Tuljapurkar predicted that the lifespan boom will be confined to wealthy countries, where citizens can afford anti-aging technology and governments can afford to sponsor scientific research. This disparity complicates the current debate over access to healthcare, as the rich become increasingly distanced from the poor, not only in quality but length of life.

Tuljapurkar warned that the distribution of anti-aging technologies is likely to be in the hands of companies that have a history of focusing solely on profit rather than the imperative to distribute medicines to those who need them most.

"Big pharmaceutical companies have a well-established track record of being very difficult when it comes to making things available to those who can't pay for them," he said.

If anti-aging technologies are distributed in the unchecked free market, "it's entirely likely to me that we'll wind up with permanent global underclasses, countries that will get locked into today's mortality conditions," Tuljapurkar said. As the gap widens and rich countries continue to invest in anti-aging technologies, the developed world may become increasingly less willing to disseminate the technology to other nations, he said: "If that happens, you get negative feedback, a vicious circle. Those countries that get locked out stay locked out."

Medical Technologies Around the World

An example of this inequality, Tuljapurkar said, is the lack of availability of AIDS antiretrovirals in Africa. Although these medications are widely available in the West, they are out of reach for many African patients, who make up more than 60 percent the world's AIDS cases. "If we can't deal with AIDS in Africa, the chance that we'll be able to deliver these anti-aging technologies to other nations is pretty slim," he said.

In the final analysis, Tuljapurkar stressed the need for scientists and policymakers alike to confront the full environmental and sociological implications of anti-aging technologies, with an awareness of the potential costs and challenges in addition to the benefits.

"What we've tended to do historically with medical advances is to take the reasonable position that we *should* implement everything that comes along," Tuljapurkar said. "However, we are now approaching a stage where it's necessary to look at the implications before we rush in—at least so we can prepare ourselves. We need to confront the prospect of inequality head-on, instead of waiting 10 years and then saying, 'What a surprise!'"

Organizations to Contact

AARP
601 E Street NW, Washington, DC   20049
(800) 424-3410
e-mail: member@aarp.org
Web site: www.aarp.org

AARP, formerly known as the American Association of Retired Persons, is a nonpartisan association that seeks to improve the aging experience for all Americans. It is committed
to the preservation of Social Security and Medicare. AARP
publishes the magazine *Modern Maturity* and the newsletter
AARP Bulletin. Issue statements and congressional testimony
can be found at the Web site.

Alliance for Aging Research
2021 K Street NW, Suite 305, Washington, DC   20006
(202) 293-2856 • fax: (202) 785-8574
e-mail: info@agingresearch.org
Web site: www.agingresearch.org

The Alliance for Aging Research is a nonprofit organization
that works to accelerate the pace of medical discoveries to improve the universal human experience of aging and health.
The organization publishes a monthly e-mail newsletter and
its Web site includes a wide array of articles, research, and up-
dates for those interested in life-extension topics.

American Geriatrics Society
350 Fifth Avenue, Suite 801, New York, NY   10118
(212) 308-1414 • fax: (212) 832-8646
e-mail: info@americangeriatrics.org
Web site: http://www.americangeriatrics.org

The American Geriatrics Society is a professional organization
of health care providers that aims to improve the health and
well-being of all older adults. AGS helps shape attitudes, poli-

cies, and practices regarding health care for older people. The society's publications include the book *The American Geriatrics Society's Complete Guide to Aging and Health*, the magazines *Journal of the American Geriatrics Society* and *Annals of Long-Term Care: Clinical Care and Aging*, and *AGS Newsletter*.

American Society on Aging
833 Market Street, Suite 511, San Francisco, CA   94103-1824
(415) 974-9600 • fax: (415) 974-0300
e-mail: info@asaging.org
Web site: www.asaging.org

The American Society on Aging is an organization of health care and social service professionals, researchers, educators, businesspeople, senior citizens, and policy makers that is concerned with all aspects of aging and works to enhance the well-being of older individuals. Its publications include the bimonthly newspaper *Aging Today* and the quarterly journal *Generations*.

Cato Institute
1000 Massachusetts Avenue NW
Washington, DC   20001-5403
(202) 842-0200 • fax: (202) 842-3490
e-mail: cato@cato.org
Web site: www.cato.org

The Cato Institute is a libertarian public-policy research foundation dedicated to limiting the control of government and protecting individual liberties. The Cato Institute publishes the magazines *Regulation* and *Cato Journal* and the online publication *Cato Unbound*.

Future of Humanity Institute
Faculty of Philosophy, University of Oxford
Oxford   OX1 1PT
   United Kingdom
01865 286279 • fax: 01865 286983
Web site: www.fhi.ox.ac.uk

The Future of Humanity Institute is a multidisciplinary research institute at the University of Oxford in England. The Institute's work centers on how anticipated technological developments may affect the human condition in fundamental ways—and how humans can better understand, evaluate, and respond to radical change. The institute publishes a monthly newsletter, and its Web site publishes the daily blog *Overcoming Bias*. The site also features research papers funded by the institute as well as other readings on the ethics and consequences of life enhancement and life extension.

Institute for Ethics and Emerging Technologies

Williams 229B, Trinity College, 300 Summit Street
Hartford, CT 06106
(860) 297-2376
e-mail: director@ieet.org
Web site: www.ieet.org

The nonprofit Institute for Ethics and Emerging Technologies was founded by philosopher Nick Bostrom and bioethicist James Hughes. The organization advocates a responsible, constructive approach to emerging human-enhancement technologies, encourages public policies for their safe and equitable use, and works to cultivate academic, professional, and popular appreciation about their impacts. In addition to offering a variety of prolongevity articles and research on its Web site, the institute publishes a series of white papers by notable names in the field, a weekly newsletter, frequent podcasts, and a daily blog.

International Federation on Ageing

425 Viger Avenue West, Suite 520, Montréal, Québec
  H2Z 1X2
(514) 396-3358 • fax: (514) 396-3378
e-mail: ifa@citenet.net
Web site: www.ifa-fiv.org

The International Federation on Ageing is a private nonprofit organization that brings together over 150 associations that represent or serve older people in 54 nations. IFA is committed to ensuring the dignity and empowerment of older persons. It publishes the quarterly journal *Ageing International* and a monthly newsletter for its members, *Intercom.*

Longevity Meme
e-mail: longevitymeme@longevitymeme.org
Web site: www.longevitymeme.org

The Longevity Meme is a nonprofit organization that encourages the development of medical technologies, lifestyles, and other means that will help people live comfortably, healthily and capably for as long as they desire, well beyond the current limits of mortality. The organization's goal is to ensure that the means and potentials of healthy life extension become commonly accepted throughout the world. The Longevity Meme Web site includes articles on longevity activism and advocacy, medical and scientific developments, and healthy living for older adults. It publishes a weekly e-mail newsletter that features commentary, news, and opinion pieces on healthy life-extension topics. Back issues are archived online. The Longevity Meme Web site also features the daily blog *Fight Aging!*

Methuseleh Foundation
P.O. Box 1143, Lorton, VA   22079-1143
(202) 306-0989
e-mail: main@methuselahfoundation.org
Web site: www.mfoundation.org

Founded by radical life-extension scientist Aubrey de Grey, the Methuselah Foundation is a nonprofit organization working to find a cure for age-related disease. The organization funds the Methuselah Mouse Prize (Mprize), a multimillion-dollar competitive research prize for the successful extension of healthy lifespan in the laboratory mouse. It also funds SENS Research, a group of detailed research proposals for repairing all known forms of aging-related damage to the human body. The group's Web site offers a wide variety of scientific articles and research papers concerning radical life extension and the biomedical advances that seek to make it a reality. The Web site publishes a daily Methuseleh Foundation blog and provides numerous links to other prolongevity blogs and online resources.

National Council on Aging
300 D Street SW, Suite 801, Washington, DC   20024
(202) 479-1200 • fax: (202) 479-0735
e-mail: info@ncoa.org
Web site: www.ncoa.org

The National Council on Aging (NCOA) is an association of organizations and professionals dedicated to promoting the dignity, self-determination, well-being, and contributions of older people. It advocates business practices, societal attitudes, and public polices that promote vital aging. NCOA's quarterly magazine, *Journal of the National Council on the Aging*, provides tools and insights for community service organizations.

President's Council on Bioethics
1425 New York Avenue NW, Suite C100
Washington, DC   20005
(202) 296-4669
e-mail: info@bioethics.gov
Web site: www.bioethics.gov

The President's Council on Bioethics is a group of individuals appointed by U.S. President George W. Bush to advise his administration on bioethics. Established on November 28, 2001, by executive order, the council is directed to "advise the President on bioethical issues that may emerge as a consequence of advances in biomedical science and technology." The council conducts research into a wide array of biomedical issues, including age retardation, life enhancement, and life extension. Reports on these topics are archived on the council's Web site and include the paper "Age-Retardation: Scientific Possibilities and Moral Challenges" and the transcript of the speech "Beyond Therapy: Ageless Bodies," given by then-chairman Leon

Kass in 2003. The council also publishes its material in book form, including the 2008 title *Human Dignity and Bioethics: Essays Commissioned by the President's Council on Bioethics.*

U.S. Administration on Aging (AOA)
330 Independence Avenue SW, Washington, DC 20201
(202) 619-0724 • fax: (202) 357-3555
e-mail: aoainfo@aoa.gov
Web site: www.aoa.dhhs.gov

The U.S. AOA works with a number of organizations, senior centers, and local service providers to help older people remain independent. It also works to protect the rights of the elderly, prevent crime and violence against older people, and investigate health care fraud. AOA's publications include fact sheets on issues such as age discrimination, elder abuse, and Alzheimer's disease. Additional publications are available through AOA's National Aging Information Center.

Bibliography

Books

Damien Broderick   *The Last Mortal Generation: How Science Will Alter Our Lives in the 21st Century.* London: New Holland Publishers, 2000.

Aubrey de Grey and Michael Rae   *Ending Aging: The Rejuvenation Breakthroughs That Could Reverse Human Aging in Our Lifetime.* New York: St. Martin's Press, 2007.

Stephen Hall   *Merchants of Immortality: Chasing the Dream of Human Life Extension.* New York: Mariner Books, 2004.

John Harris   "Intimations of Immortality—The Ethics and Justice of Life Extending Therapies." In M. Freeman, ed., *Current Legal Problems.* Oxford, United Kingdom: Oxford University Press, 2003.

Immortality Institute   *The Scientific Conquest of Death: Essays on Infinite Lifespans.* Buenos Aires: Libros en Red, 2004.

Glenn McGee   *The New Immortality: Science and Speculation About Extending Life Forever.* Albany, CA: Berkeley Hills Books, 2002.

Harry Moody   *Aging: Concepts and Controversies,*
                       3rd edition. Thousand Oaks, CA:
                       Pine Forge, 2000.

Stephen Post and   *The Fountain of Youth: Cultural*
Robert Binstock,   *Scientific and Ethical Perspectives on a*
eds.   *Biomedical Goal.* Oxford, United
                       Kingdom: Oxford University Press,
                       2004.

James Schultz and   *Aging Nation: The Economics and*
Robert Binstock   *Politics of Growing Older in America.*
                       Westport, CT: Praeger, 2006.

Periodicals

David Bloom and   "The Health and Wealth of Nations,"
David Canning   *Science* 287, February 18, 2000.

Nick Bostrom   "Recent Developments in the Ethics,
                       Science, and Politics of
                       Life-Extension," *Aging Horizons,*
                       Autumn/Winter 2005.

John Davis   "Collective Suttee: Is It Just to
                       Develop Life Extension if It Will Not
                       Be Possible to Provide It to
                       Everyone?" *Annals of the New York*
                       Academy of Sciences 1019, June 2004.

John Davis   "The Prolongevists Speak Up: The
                       Life-Extension Ethics Session at the
                       10th Annual Congress of the
                       International Association of
                       Biomedical Gerontology," *The*
                       American Journal of Bioethics 4,
                       December 2004.

Davis Gems   "Is More Life Always Better? The New Biology of Aging and the Meaning of Life," *Hastings Center Report* 33, July/August 2003.

Leonard Hayflick   "'Anti-Aging' Is an Oxymoron," *Journals of Gerontology* 59, no. 6, June 2004.

Leon Kass   "Ageless Bodies, Happy Souls: Biotechnology and the Pursuit of Perfection," presented at the Ethics and Public Policy Center, Washington, DC, January 9, 2003.

Leon Kass   "Beyond Therapy: Biotechnology and the Pursuit of Human Improvement," presented as speech to the President's Council on Bioethics, January 2003.

Michael Mason   "One for the Ages: A Prescription That May Extend Life," *New York Times*, October 31, 2006.

Sherwin Nuland   "Do You Want to Live Forever?" *Technology Review*, Massachusetts Institute of Technology, February 2005.

James Oeppen and James Vaupel   "Broken Limits to Life Expectancy," *Science* 296, May 10, 2002.

Jay Olshansky   "Can We Justify Efforts to Slow the Rate of Aging in Humans?" presentation before the annual meeting of the Gerontological Society of America, 2003.

Jay Olshansky, Leonard Hayflick, et al.   "Position Statement on Human Aging," *Journals of Gerontology* 57, no. 8, August 2002.

Martien Pijnenburg   "Who Wants to Live Forever? Three Arguments Against Extending the Human Lifespan," *Journal of Medical Ethics* 33, no. 10, October 2007.

Public Agenda   "The Science of Aging Gracefully: Scientists and the Public Talk About Aging Research," Alliance for Aging Research and the American Federation for Aging Research, 2005.

Gregory Stock, Daniel Callahan, and Aubrey de Grey   "The Ethics of Life Extension," *Rejuvenation Research*, September 1, 2007.

Index